The
Body Map
Supplemental

How I Reversed Type II Diabetes and What I Learned Along the Way

T. M. Cocklin
CSL, CCF

The Body Map: *Supplemental*
How I Reversed Type II Diabetes
and What I learned along the way.

© 2020 Worlds of Wonder Publishing
Dallas, Texas

ISBN-13: 978-0-9966317-4-7

Cover Design - Tim Cocklin, Photos from Shutterstock.com

Address all correspondence to:
tim@worldsofwonderpublishing.com

OTHER BOOKS
By Tim Cocklin

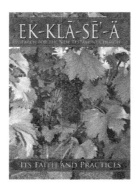

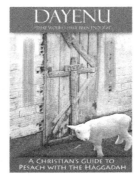

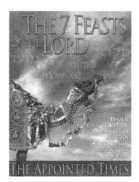

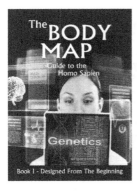

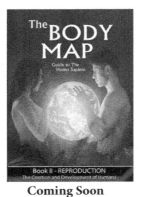

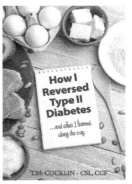

Coming Soon

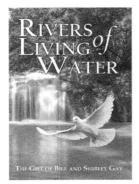

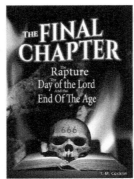

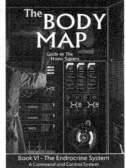

Coming Soon

The information in this book is **NOT** to be taken as advice or a prescription for overcoming diabetes, it is for education purposes only. I am not a Medical Doctor. Please check with a Medical professional before starting any health regiment.

Appendix B has a short list of Medical professionals who understand the issues and have the authority to help you with your issue.

"Let food be your medicine."
Hippocrates

"Good food needs no medicine,
bad food does."
Robert H. Lustig, M.D.
American pediatric endocrinologist
University of California, San Francisco

STOP!
Take this quiz before reading the book
Circle [T] True or [F] False:

1. [T] [F] Eating foods high in saturated fats, Like butter, and eggs will cause you to get fat & increase your chances of a heart attack.
2. [T] [F] High cholesterol causes heart disease & diabetes.
3. [T] [F] To be healthy we must lower LDL cholesterol.
4. [T] [F] To permanently lose weight eat less and exercise more.
5. [T] [F] Statin drugs will solve the problems caused by high cholesterol.
6. [T] [F] Follow the USDA food pyramid for guaranteed good health.
7. [T] [F] A calorie is a calorie, all calories are the same.
8. [T] [F] Diabetes is a Chronic disease and must be treated with Insulin
9. [T] [F] Raw cow's milk (unpasteurized) will make you sick.
10. [T] [F] Margarine better for you than butter.
11. [T] [F] Vegetable oils come from a variety of vegetables.
12. [T] [F] Doctors get a significant education in nutritional science.
13. [T] [F] We need carbohydrates to maintain good health.
14. [T] [F] If you are athletic you must have carbohydrates for energy.
15. [T] [F] Fruit juices are essential for good health.
16. [T] [F] Foods that have the heart healthy designation from the America Heart Association have been proven to be beneficial to health.
17. [T] [F] Eggs: Eat the whites only, the yoke is full of bad cholestrol.
18. [T] [F] Eating a low fat diet rich in carbohydrates is best.
19. [T] [F] Strenuous exercise is necessary for weight loss.
20. [T] [F] Your arteries get clogged with fat just like when you pour grease down your drain, causing heart attacks.
21. [T] [F] A vegetarian diet is best for complete health
22. [T] [F] Animal fats cause cancer and heart disease.
23. [T] [F] Coconut Oil or Palm Kernel Oil both cause heart disease.
24. [T] [F] Soy foods protect against many types of cancer.
25. [T] [F] To avoid heart disease, use margarine instead of butter.
26. [T] [F] The brain requires glucose that only comes from carbohydrates.
27. [T] [F] The best way to lose weight is low fat and less calories
28. [T] [F] A large percentage of people who die from heart attack or stroke have a high level of LDL-cholesterol.
29. [T] [F] HDL is good cholesterol and LDL is bad cholesterol.
30. [T] [F] Statin drugs significantly reduce death by heart attack.

We have followed the advice of the medical community which told us for optimal health: One, Eat less and exercise more, and two follow a diet of low-fat rich in carbohydrates like whole grains, fruits and vegetables and limit saturated fats.

What has happened since we followed their advice from the late 1970s?
Article · May 2016 Richard Lear - Brown University

The Root Cause in the dramatic rise of Chronic Disease
See discussions, stats, and author profiles for this publication at:
https://www.researchgate.net/publication/303673576

"The annual economic burden of just thirty-six fast-growing chronic diseases tracked in this paper is more than $**2.77 trillion**. This is more than 70% of the current annual federal budget. With increased public awareness, coupled with a federal government commitment to dedicated research on the mechanisms and cures for the Diseases of Civilization, this cost to society can be reduced to a fraction – by simply acting on the knowledge we already have."

"While the major health threats of the 20th century - cardiovascular disease, infectious disease and cancer - are barely growing, at least 36 chronic diseases and disorders have more than doubled in the past generation. Twenty have more than tripled. Many of these new age diseases were unknown until the 1980s. Here is a sampling of the growth in prevalence of diseases and disorders"

Autism (2,094%)	*Alzheimer's* (299%)
COPD (148%)	**diabetes (305%)**
Sleep apnea (430%)	celiac disease (1,111%)
ADHD (819%)	asthma (142%)
Depression (280%)	*youth bipolar disease*
(10,833%)	
Osteoarthritis (449%)	lupus (787%)
Inflammatory bowel (120%)	chronic fatigue (11,027%)
fibromyalgia (7,727%)	multiple sclerosis (117%)
hypothyroidism (702%)."	

Five syndromes on the list (in italic) are related to the brain! It is my belief that these issues have to do with highly processed foods, additives like extra sugar in many forms, chemicals in our environment and the medical profession's response to the issues.

If you answered false to all the questions on page IV, you are correct, you have not fallen for the misguidance and faulty information of the health gurus. If you read the rest of this book, you will find out why all the answers are false. We have all been subject to policies of health organizations, drug companies and food manufacturers who have proven to be the cause of a tremendous amount of pain and suffering! This must change; the costs are mounting exponentially and the number of people subject to ill-health from following bad advice is staggering!

WARNING

What you are about to read is way out of the mainstream of current medical practice. What you will discover is that we have been following the pied piper of bad advice. We have a health crisis of biblical proportions. The directives we have been given have resulted in a pandemic of obesity and ill health. If you show this to your medical professional, they will likely "freak out" and give you all the reasons why it is wrong. However, I am proof that you can overcome obesity and diabetes without drugs, much to the displeasure of food and drug companies.

Much of what we have been sold as health is, in fact, counter to the actual facts. For instance: You may believe that eating fat will make you fat! The exact opposite is true as are many other beliefs, I will illustrate in this book.

"The poor quality of medical research is widely acknowledged, yet disturbingly the leaders of the medical profession seem only minimally concerned about the problems and make no apparent efforts to find a solution."

- Richard Smith – editor of the BMJ.

**A special thanks to
Shirley Gay and Cindy Cocklin
for correcting the textual mistakes
I made while writing**

"If eating saturated fat caused heart disease and weight gain, then eliminating those fats should have resulted in a decline in heart disease and an increase in weight loss. But look around you. That's not what happened!"

- Dr. Mary Enig and Sally Fallon
Eat Fat Lose Fat. Page 21

"Back in the MI (myocardial infarction- heart attack) free days before 1920, the fats were butter and lard and I think that we would all benefit from the kind of diet that we had at a time when no one had ever heard the word corn oil."

– Dr. Dudley White speaking at an American Heart Association fund raiser in 1956.

Content

My story on Dietdoctor.com
https://www.dietdoctor.com/keto-success-story-i-can-tell-you-it-   has-been-a-godsend-to-me

NOTE:

If you find terms that are not clearly defined, or topics that are not understandable, please send me an email at:
diabetes@worldsofwonderpublishing.com
I will include more detail in the next update of the book.

Section 1

Beginning
The Journey to
Health

"We define the problem not the symptom. When you define the problem you get different answers than when you define the symptom"

- Patrick Theut
Reversing Calcification Episode 21
The Fat Emperor - Ivor Cummins

Put another way:

When the medical profession only focuses on symptoms, they look for ways to alleviate the symptom also known as "treating the disease", usually by drugs. Addressing symptoms will never cure the underlying cause. You must find out what caused the issue in the first place.

Case in point: Dealing with blood sugar levels by prescribing drugs has never prevented or cured diabetes! It only prolongs the misery and suffering. The current approach to treating the disease is why diabetes is a progressive disease, those diagnosed with Type II will need more and more drugs to deal with increasing blood sugar levels until they deal with the original cause of high blood sugar.

- Tim Cocklin

I

INTRODUCTION

> "If we all worked on the assumption that what is accepted as true is really true, there would be little hope of advance."
> - Orville Wright

The human body is complex beyond our comprehension. I have made a study of the Homo Sapien physiology, and I am researching and writing a series of 12 books, which describe in detail what I have learned about the various parts of the body (The Body Map Series). There are many factors, which will keep us healthy or make us sick. There are hormones, organs, chemistry and a myriad of other factors that keep us alive, but mistreat it, or expose it to a harmful environment, and the body will begin to break down. Each cell in the body is an amazing factory operating 24 hours a day, taking in nutrients, creating energy, exporting waste. Exposure to harmful chemicals in the environment and in our food contribute to the breakdown. We are still learning things about ourselves and how the body functions. We were created to function in a specific way, if we feed our bodies with the suitable fuel, get the proper amount of sleep, live as stress free as we can, get a sufficient amount of exercise and stay away from harmful chemicals, we can remain healthy. However, very few of us live in utopia these days. We don't always get the sleep we need; we live in a high-stress world; food companies remove God-given nutrition replacing it with man-made concoctions and harmful chemicals are dumped into our environment among other things. The medical community is quick to prescribe drugs to relieve symptoms but are not always trained to address the cause of the illness. If you are not genetically hampered in some way there is hope. We must therefore, find a way to overcome the deleterious effects of our world if we are to have good health and a long healthy life.

I have discovered a way to reverse my diabetes through diet alone. When I researched why I had high blood sugar and stopped trying to cover up the symptom with drugs, something miraculous happened; my diabetes disappeared. Keep in mind, the body is too complex for a "one thing fixes all" approach to health. My research has led me in countless directions. Like an onion, I keep pealing back the layers only to find another layer beneath it. Just when I think, I have the answer to overall good health, I find some other factor, which affects our health. I hope that this book will reveal some of the reasons we get ill, how to avoid them and point the way to information and resources that will put you on your way to vibrant health.

However, I am *ANGRY, INFURIATED AND FUMING;* we have been deceived! We have been lied to by a self-serving and arrogant food, drug, political, educational and nutritional health community. You will find in the history of medicine that the intellectual arrogance of medical "professionals and experts" rejected change in their thinking, making progress almost impossible. We would not have the cures that we have today if courageous men did not persist in their beliefs. I don't blame the nutritionist or doctors; they have been indoctrinated to believe the prevarication. The guidelines presented in the late 70s were NOT based on any scientific study. As a matter of fact, it is said that some of the trials used to prove animal fats (saturated fats) and cholesterol were the cause of heart disease, actually used margarine and vegetable (seed) oils in their testing. These are substances which actually cause problems, we will discuss why later in the book.

I have read more than 12 books now in my search of how to reverse type II diabetes; Virtually all of them buy into the low-fat, cholesterol deception. All the books I could find follow the advice of "the authorities and experts" that suggest keeping total cholesterol under 200, as if cholesterol is the cause of ill health. All the research I have done and my own experience would call that "bunk"! Others get caught up in the energy-in/energy-out scenario. This leads to the recommendation that all you need to do is eat less and exercise more, the calorie deficit plan. In the long run, this approach does not work. Some suggest that carbohydrates are necessary for good health, and the brain requires the glucose that comes from them. This is simply not true! Keytones, from good fats, are a very excellent source of fuel for the brain. There is **NO** requirement in the body for carbohydrates! I am not saying you shouldn't enjoy them, but in moderation.

Diabetes is a chronic and progressive disease, and the symptoms will get worse over time... *if you follow the advice of experts and doctors like I did.*

Reminder: I am researching the issues; I am not a licensed doctor and do not practice medicine. You need to contact a practitioner who has the right to diagnose and treat your issue, see appendix B for a list of practitioners. Nothing in this book should be taken as medical advice.

Introduction

> "The lower limit of dietary carbohydrate compatible with life apparently is zero, provided that adequate amounts of protein and fat are consumed. However, the amount of dietary carbohydrate that provides for optimal health in humans is unknown. There are traditional populations that ingested a high fat, high protein diet containing only a minimal amount of carbohydrate for extended periods of time (the Massai), and in some cases for a lifetime after infancy (Alaska and Greenland Natives, Inuits, and Pampas indigenous people) (Du Bois, 1928; Paul Heinbecker, 1928).

Everyone who I have talked to tell the same story: "I did not get better but steadily got worse and had to take more and more drugs." The lipid hypothesis which states that high-cholesterol causes blocked arteries and other diseases, from eating saturated fats, eggs and red meat is misleading at best and a lie at worst. I can site numerous examples that prove that point of view wrong, not withstanding my own experience! I do not generally buy into conspiracy theories, but there has to be a reason why, after decades of failure, we see an increase in diabetes and obesity following their advice not a decrease. To verify that, just look at pictures of groups of people before the 1970s, you will find obesity and exception rather than the rule. Could it be that they are more concerned with profit than health? What the experts recommend is clearly **NOT** working and has not worked for decades! If I had continued taking their drugs and eating their recommended diet, I am sure I would be dead by now. However, I stopped taking their advice, and I have reversed, what they call irreversible. This is my story; I hope it will inspire you to do your own research and seek help from doctors who have a proven track record of reversing obesity and type II diabetes.

I will warn you that there is no one-size-fits-all diet. What works for one may not work for another. However, there are general truths that will work for everyone. You must take your health into your own hands. Start with advice from those medical professionals who have a track record of actually reversing diabetes in the long run. Experiment with different ideas until you discover what works for you. I took one approach and reversed my diabetes and lost weight; however, my wife (who was not diabetic) did not lose weight as dramatically as I did. We are experimenting with different approaches to help her lose the weight she wants to lose... once and for all.

There is no one "PERFECT diet," your experience is unique. As you start your own journey, keep in mind that diet is only one aspect of health, a major one of course, but there are other factors to consider. Stress, poor sleep habits, endocrine disruptors, your current epigenetic markers (we will discuss these later) drugs you may be taking currently and your level of physical activity.

The Senate in 1977, led by Senator George McGovern was told by scientists that the recommendations they were making were not adequately studied, and they wanted more research before the announcements of the guidelines were given to the American public. McGovern said, "I would only argue that Senators don't have the luxury that a research scientist does of waiting until every last shred of evidence is in." As a result, we have all been the victims of their rush to judgment and the grand failed experiment. We have all suffered enormously in terms of bad health and the sky rocketing cost to deal with their dreadful advice. This rush to make recommendations on health was a result of biased information and politics. Now the food and drug companies have had decades to entrench themselves into the fabric of the U.S. and other cultures around the world with devastating effects! This hypothesis was finally released in 1980 as Dietary Guidelines for Americans, and we have all suffered for it and continue to suffer under its devastating effects.

I was slowly being murdered, yes I said murdered, by prescription drugs, fast food and a lot of very bad advice. Thank God, I took my health into my own hands and did the research and started listening to those who have a track record of reversing disease. What the government and medical community have been telling us about cholesterol, and saturated fats are *DEAD* wrong. When I stopped listening to the false statements, and went on a totally different diet, one they told me would kill me, I began to get healthy, and I lost weight. My blood sugar and blood pressure normalized along with a lot of other health markers without the side effects of prescription drugs! And yet in July of 2019 the doctor I went to suggested lowering cholesterol by using a statin and recommended a low-fat diet! I will expound on that as we go.

> **"Don't listen to the voices that sold you the diet that made you sick in the first place" - Dr. Peter Ballerstedt**

If your premise is flawed, your recommendations will be wrong! Everything I have read and studied, reveals that it is NOT cholesterol or saturated fat that cause heart disease, obesity and diabetes. There is a cause for all these diseases but not what we have been told. I have heard some say that it is like blaming fire fighters for the fire, since they always show up when there is a fire. So too, cholesterol is present when there is a growing abnormality in the arteries, but cholesterol is NOT the cause! It is inflammation and other factors like the damage from free radicals.

The American Heart Association, National Institutes of Health, The USDA and other organizations all recommend a diet low in saturated fats and cholesterol (now suggesting less than 7% saturated fat). The research I have found and my own experience show that the premise is based on bias and bad science. You will see that the recommendations have not lived up to the promise. In fact, things have gotten much worse and are continuing the trend to get even more problematic as people follow their recommendations. All you need to do is look at the sponsors of these organizations to see where the influence is coming from today.

> "For people who need to lower their cholesterol, the American Heart Association recommends reducing saturated fat to no more than **5 to 6 percent of total daily calories**. For someone eating 2,000 calories a day, that's about 11 to 13 grams of saturated fat".
>
> - American Heart Association (accessed 8/2/2019)

This book was written to share information and sources, which have been helpful to me on my journey to reversing diabetes and obesity. For everyone who has health issues, this information cannot guarantee improved health, but it is the best counsel I have found for losing weight, gaining and sustaining health. I suggest that you do your own research and come to your personal conclusion and check with the doctors listed in appendix B. This book has plenty of resources for doing your personal research. To me, the best evidence for truth is actual experience not hearsay from biased sources. Today, doctors are trained to identify a problem and treat it with a regiment of drugs or programs that do not work in the long run; I speak from experience.

After following the advice of the *Dietary Guidelines for Americans*, obesity and disease have increased dramatically! It would be insane to continue to follow these guidelines off the cliff to your increasing poor health or even death! Not to mention the enormous cost associated with the standard American diet (S.A.D.) However, if you are like me, I did not know what I know now and no medical professional whom I have dealt with did either. Medical doctors are trained to recognize a symptom and afterwards prescribe a treatment, usually with drugs. Many times the drug sales person is the one who educates the doctor on the latest drug and next leaves plenty of samples to give to their patients. Thank God, more and more cardiologists are rejecting the current example and are choosing to do the right thing for their patients.

According to Healthline in an article on:
https://www.healthline.com/health/leading-causes-of-death
Written by Kimberly Holland and medically reviewed by Deborah Weatherspoon, PhD, RN, CRNA on November 1, 2018.

The 12 leading causes of death are:

1. **Heart disease** - deaths per year: 635,260
2. **Cancer** - deaths per year: 598,038
3. **Accidents** (unintentional injuries) deaths per year: 161,374
4. **Chronic lower respiratory diseases** deaths per year: 154,596
5. **Stroke** - deaths per year: 142,142
6. **Alzheimer's disease** - deaths per year: 116,103
7. **Diabetes** - deaths per year: 80,058
8. **Influenza and pneumonia** - deaths per year: 51,537
9. **Kidney disease** - deaths per year: 50,046
10. **Suicide** - deaths per year: 44,965
11. **Septicemia** - deaths per year: 38,940
12. **Chronic liver disease and cirrhosis** - deaths per year: 38,170

Other than accidents and suicide, it is my belief that these causes of death can be lowered by proper lifestyle and nutrition. NOT by drugs and ill-advised recommendations by current methods that have proven to be false. I hope to provide you with the information and resources to improve your health and keep you from the maladies above.

Unfortunately, doctors are generally held captive to the "Standard of Care" which we will discuss in the chapter on the history of medicine. This means they are held to standards which may be outdated and not helpful but are dictated by the medical establishment. But, cross the line and the doctor is subject to losing their status or license.

This is the story of my journey to real health. I will quote many medical and research experts who educated me along the way. Most of these doctors and researchers go against the widely accepted advice of U.S. Government recommendations, which were formulated in the 1950s by faulty science and propagated by food and drug companies. The guideline opponents are courageous men and women who dare take on the medical establishment with proof of their findings. Plus there is a growing number like myself who have taken a different approach to health and have won.

We have a health crisis of biblical proportions caused by bad science and biased research studies. The cost of health care is skyrocketing, debilitating and fatal diseases are on the rise. There seems to be no answer. There is, however, an answer if only the experts and authorities listen to real evidence-based medicine and not special-interest groups. The naysayers will try to dismiss what the evidence clearly shows, but there are those like myself who rebel against their errant advice. There are multitudes which, like myself, who have reversed the effects of a bad diet and are on the way to good health. Obesity, diabetes and heart disease are now in the rear-view mirror for many of us. Say what they may, there are multitudes that have come before me and have done what I have done and are perfectly healthy today.

Anyone who wants to change the status quo will get negative push back from the establishment. The attack from the establishment is typically not against the ideas that are presented but against the person who made the audacious suggestion. ...I will not hold my breath waiting for the change, as they say, "you can't change city hall." To get to the bottom of the issue "Follow the money"! You will find, when you get there, how companies have been in pushing their products regardless of the adverse consequences all in the name of profit. The tobacco industry proved that to be true by dismissing any negative suggestions and telling us that smoking is not harmful! How did that work out for us? However, food companies produce foods that the public demands with their dollars. We are still seeing the effects of the low-fat craze. I have been to multiple grocery stores trying to find chicken breasts with the skin; it is rare. Everywhere I go products tout the fact that they are "Low-fat." But, what had to be done to remove the fat? Let's take milk, for instance.

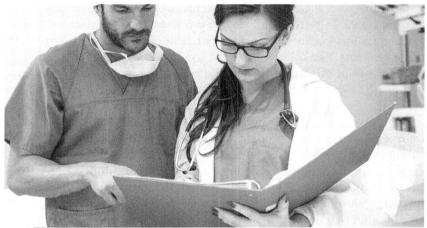

THE 12 LEADING CAUSES OF DEATH ARE:

1. HEART DISEASE - DEATHS PER YEAR:	635,260
2. CANCER - DEATHS PER YEAR:	598,038
3. ACCIDENTS (UNINTENTIONAL INJURIES) DEATHS PER YEAR:	161,374
4. CHRONIC LOWER RESPIRATORY DISEASES DEATHS PER YEAR:	154,596
5. STROKE - DEATHS PER YEAR:	142,142
6. ALZHEIMER'S DISEASE - DEATHS PER YEAR:	116,103
7. DIABETES - DEATHS PER YEAR:	80,058
8. INFLUENZA AND PNEUMONIA - DEATHS PER YEAR:	51,537
9. KIDNEY DISEASE - DEATHS PER YEAR:	50,046
10. SUICIDE - DEATHS PER YEAR:	44,965
11. SEPTICEMIA - DEATHS PER YEAR:	38,940
12. CHRONIC LIVER DISEASE AND CIRRHOSIS - DEATHS PER YEAR:	38,170

HTTPS://WWW.HEALTHLINE.COM/HEALTH/LEADING-CAUSES-OF-DEATH
WRITTEN BY KIMBERLY HOLLAND AND MEDICALLY REVIEWED BY DEBORAH WEATHERSPOON, PhD, RN, CRNA ON November 1, 2018.

Introduction ■■■■■■■■■■
What is wrong with skim milk?

The first thing done to make skim milk is to spin the whole milk in a centrifuge and thereby separating the fat molecules. The issue with this process is that vitamins A and D are fat soluble, these are lost in the process. *Strike 1*. The taste is not good. My nephew's mother (who actually has a nursing degree) innocently thought her son should only drink skim or 2% milk because she was taught that fat is bad. When he came to our house, he drank several glasses because we had whole milk, he remarked how good it tasted. In virtually all fat-free products, the manufacture must add sugar in some form to make it palatable. *Strike 2*. The texture of fat-free products, like skim milk, is not good and shelf life is reduced. Because of the poor texture and reduced shelf life, the manufacture puts in surfactants (to lower the surface tension between two liquids) and emulsifiers (interfaces the conflicting components of food like water and oil) like mono and diglycerides (food manufacturers typically use monoglycerides and diglycerides to extend a product's shelf life). *Strike 3 (you're out)*. According to the Weston Price Foundation "Powered skim milk, is a source of dangerous oxidized cholesterol and neurotoxic amino acids." The manufacture takes a natural food, strips out all the nutrition and then adds back a lot of man-made concoctions to make it palatable and give it the perceived notion that it is healthy when, in fact, it is not. Why? All because we are told that saturated fat is bad! Three strikes and you are out!

Why should we consume whole Grass-Fed, UNPASTEURIZED milk? According to the Weston Price Foundation: "nutrients like vitamin A,D,E, and K are greatest from cows eating green grass, but are diminished when the cows are fed commercial feed." ..."Soy meal contains thyroid-depressing estrogen components." They go on to say: "Pasteurization destroys enzymes denatures anti-microbial and immune-stimulating components, kills beneficial bacteria, promotes pathogens, and destroys vitamins C, B6 and B12... " For more detail, please visit www.realmilk.com and www. westonaprice.com.

If you have ever talked to a person who has struggled with a weight problem for a long time, you will hear a reply like: "I have tried everything; I lose the weight, but the weight only comes back." This is universal, everyone I have spoken to have a story similar to the one I just quoted. Every year we hear of a new diet which is long on the promise but short on delivery. For the most part, every diet plan has failed to some degree. Why? It is my contention that the premises of these diets are all wrong. Especially those that say: "Eat less and Exercise more." The truth is that it is more about what you eat than how much you exercise. I am not saying that you should not exercise, I do all the time, but it is not the best way to lose excess fat. And tests plus my own experience has proven, that eating less slows down your metabolism even further each time you go on a low-calorie diet. There are studies that prove that fact. A popular television weight loss show of extremely obese participants prove that overtime participants experience weight gain after being on their very rigid program of diet and exercise. In order to maintain their weight, they have to eat less or regain what they have lost. Extreme low calorie and strenuous exercise will work, but only in the short run. Why? A low calorie, low-fat diet will make you hungry! Most people cannot stick with it. The more you diet this way the harder it gets, because your metabolism slows down so you have to eat less and less.

If you try to live by the infamous food pyramid recommended by the health industry, you will find that it does not work in practice for people with long-term weight problems. Not everyone has an issue with weight. However, I can predict that if you go on a strict low calorie/low-fat diet over time your metabolism will be affected! Any weight loss will quickly return and most times you will gain even more weight. This gain comes back because your metabolism has slowed.

It is my hope that this book will enlighten you and explain why the food pyramid generally does not work. Since the introduction of highly processed foods, we have become more obese and have seen an ever-increasing number of chronic and fatal diseases. Think of the low-fat craze? People thought that fat causes you to get fat and eating food low in fat would not cause you to gain weight. The result was catastrophic! People eating low-fat foods became fatter. Notwithstanding, go into to any store, even health-food stores, and notice all the products that proclaim the fact they are low fat! While you are looking at the food content label, look at how much sugar is added, you will be amazed how many products have added sugar, although the sugar may be hidden under a different names. I checked the ingredients of a sausage product that said it had no sugar. Many times you will find that the second ingredient is corn syrup. Corn syrup is actually worse than sugar because fructose can only be processed in the liver. We sill discuss this later in our chapter on Sugar: Pure, White and deadly a title of a book by John Yudkin a British doctor...

Don't forget about the Frito-lay experiment with WOW chips. These were "fat-free" and contained Olestra. Olestra was approved by the FDA for use as a food additive in 1996. The first year of the WOW product Frito-lay sold about $400 million of their products. The issue with the product is that it caused numerous problems: diarrhea, anal leakage, and other gastrointestinal problems. "You cannot fool mother nature" as the saying goes. Long term use of the product may have been catastrophic!

I saw a breakfast sausage that had added sugar and worse it had MSG (Mono-sodium Glutamate)! Why would you put sugar and MSG in sausage? Is it the low quality of the meat itself? You have to make it taste better or people won't buy it! MSG is an exotoxin which will over stimulate the brain. This man-made concoction is linked to headaches, fatigue and other poor health symptoms.

It has been said that MSG also leads to leptin resistance. Leptin is the hormone that tells your brain that you are full, more on this later. Have you ever eaten Chinese food (loaded with MSG) and wanted more and more after having eaten "enough"? See the chart on the next page (thanks to Debby Anglesey for permission to bring you this chart. See how the food manufactures hide MSG in their foods.

We have already seen the dramatic increase in diseases since the 1980s illustrated by the article by Richard Lear at Brown University earlier. I noted that at least five of these were related to the brain. The brain requires cholesterol and can produce some but not all for its needs. However, the radical oxidation and inflammation factors introduced by ingesting ill-advised foods will cause problems to grow. The cost of these debilitating diseases is staggering and should not be allowed to grow, or it will result in totally bankrupting us. Could this be the financial collapse of America? Can this pandemic be reversed? Yes, but it will take a lot of us banding together and demanding change.

From the website: https://www.msgmyth.com/hidden-names used with permission. The following substances always contain factory created free glutamate, with MSG containing 78%.

MSG	Gelatin	Calcium glutamate
Mono-sodium glutamate	Hydrolyzed Vegetable Protein	Textured Protein
Mono-potassium glutamate	Hydrolyzed Plant Protein (HPP)	Yeast Extract
Glutamate	Autolyzed Plant Protein	Yeast food or nutrient
Glutamic Acid	Sodium Caseinate	Autolyzed Yeast
Vegetable Protein Extract	Senomyx (labeled:artificial flavor)	Any hydrolyzed protein
Calcium Caseinate	Sodium caseinate	Magnesium glutamate
Mono-ammonium glutamate	Soy protein,	Whey protein, whey protein isolate
Natrium glutamate	Ajinomoto	Vestin
Anything hydrolyzed or autolyzed		

BOOK: *Battling the MSG Myth* - by Debby Anglesey

Foods that used to be nutritious are now overly processed so that all the God-given nutrients are removed and replaced with man made chemical concoctions. Foods that are labeled as heart healthy are anything but healthy. You will find, later on in this book, that companies pay to have the heart healthy label on their products.

Question: are fruit juices healthy? Remember the slogan "A day without orange juice is like a day without sunshine"? We are told that juices are healthy. You will find that when producers take out the fiber, and pasteurize it, the quality of the fruit is virtually nil. Even if you juice the fruit at home, and do not pasteurize it, by removing the fiber you have effectively taken away the one thing that God put in the fruit that will balance the amount of sugar you are about to consume. It is far better to eat the entire fruit. In any case, how many fruits does it take to make an eight oz glass of juice? It generally takes four oranges. I would guess more than you would eat at one time. Drinking juiced fruit means you are then drinking concentrated fructose sugar. We will show that fructose in excess will cause a number of problems. Fructose can only be processed in the liver. Excess fructose will cause a host of issues we will discuss later.

Many of the so called "heart health foods" are loaded with sugar and refined carbohydrates. It is a proven fact that sugar causes many issues in the human body, including but certainly not limited to tooth decay. We will address the deleterious effects of sugar later in another chapter. If we consume the same food they did 100 years ago, mostly unprocessed and raw, I believe our health statistics would improve dramatically. Those who have studied cultures where the modern diet has not infected their lifestyle, you will find a healthy population free from most of the modern diseases we suffer in the United States. Additionally, we do not know the long-term effects of these chemical additives and genetically modified organisms (GMO) in our food supply. The FDA has deemed them safe, but I am not convinced that they are safe. The growing ill health of Americans and any society that takes on the Standard American Diet (S.A.D.) is proof that they are not acceptable. (see *Seeds of Deception & GMO* - Jeffrey Smith)

Let's say you were going bald and someone suggested the combing your hair backwards 100 times a day would regrow your hair, you would most likely try it. When that technique does not work, how likely are you to suggest it to other people going bald? Most of us would tell everyone that it does not work. It has been overwhelmingly proven that the "eat less/exercise more" scenarios generally do not work over time for most people, and the constantly increasing obesity and disease problem proves it. When will the medical profession quit recommending or prescribing something that does not work? The issue is that the one attempting weight loss and failing are told it is their fault, "if they only ate less and exercise more" or "you must not be following the guidelines correctly." However, every doctor and nutritionist I have been to suggest that very thing. It has not worked, THERE HAS TO BE ANOTHER ANSWER! I believe I have found the answer for better health at least for myself. There is no one size fits all when it comes to health, we are all distinctive; our backgrounds are unique our genetics are different our epigenetic markers are all distinct, and our lifestyles are individual. A case in point is that my wife is on the same eating plan that I am, and yet she is not losing weight as quickly as I have. At the time, I am writing this we are still researching to find the right combination of things that will get her into a continuous fat-burning mode. There are, however, sound principles that can lead to exceptional health. The current recommendations by the medical community have not been successful at getting us to a state of good health. To find a medical professional who has a proven track record of helping people with your issue see appendix B.

"In an address to students at the Medical School, he said, "Half of what we are going to teach you is wrong, and half of it is right. Our problem is that we don't know which half is which."
- Charles Sidney Burwell - Dean of Harvard Medical School 1935-1949

"Half of what you'll learn in medical school will be shown to be either dead wrong or out of date within five years of your graduation; the trouble is that nobody can tell you which half–so the most important thing to *learn is how to learn on your own*." - Dr. David Sackett, often referred to as the "father of evidence-based medicine 1930 - 2015

Reminder: I am researching the issues; I am not a licensed doctor and do not practice medicine. You need to contact a practitioner who has the right to diagnose and treat your issue, see appendix B for a list of practitioners. Nothing in this book should be taken as medical advice.

At the time of this research, we have seen an unprecedented shutdown of the world economy. Initially, we knew very little about the covid-19 virus. Because we had no idea how the virus would spread it was wise to stop as much interaction between people as possible to hinder a global pandemic. However, as time went on we discovered that it was not as dangerous to healthy individuals as the models predicted. In reality, less than 2% of the people who contract the virus actually die from it. And the overwhelming number that die have other underlying issues like diabetes and other health issues. In many cases' people who get the virus have mild or no symptoms at all.

It is difficult to get accurate information because this event has been overly politicized. It may be some time before we know the absolute truth. Currently, we can only speculate the effect this virus has had on the health of the citizens. However, some of the suggestions by the "experts" are ridiculous at best and insane in the worst cases. Case in point: Dr. Tony Fauci said, "Americans should not shake hands, ever again."

God designed an immune system to protect us from germs, viruses and other nasty bugs. Generally speaking once you have had a virus, your body has the amazing ability to build a defense against it and will remember and have in reserve the antibodies to fight it if it attempts to infiltrate your system again.

To try to hide from all germs is a very bad idea. It is not practical for us to live in a completely antiseptic environment. At this point, I think to continue the lock down is foolish. Hopefully, common sense will prevail. We will see in the coming days.

How Blood Sugar Can Trigger a Deadly Immune Response in the Flu and Possibly COVID-19

From :
https://www.scientificamerican.com/article/how-blood-sugar-can-trigger-a-deadly-immune-response-in-the-flu-and-possibly-covid-191/
by Tanya Lewis on April 24, 2020

"Glucose metabolism plays a key role in the cytokine storm seen in influenza, and the link could have potential implications for novel coronavirus infections."

In its latest study, the team revealed, at a detailed molecular level, how a glucose metabolism pathway activated by flu infection leads to an out-of-control immune response. During such an infection, high levels of glucose in the blood cause an enzyme called O-linked β-N-acetylglucosamine transferase (OGT) to bind to, and chemically modify, IRF5 in a process known as glycosylation. This step enables another chemical modification, called ubiquitination, that leads to a cytokine inflammatory response.

"Influenza and COVID-19 infections can trigger an out-of-control immune response involving molecules called cytokines".

Note: Cytokines regulate the immune response and intervene in cell-to-cell communication. It is no wonder then that diabetics have more issues with the virus than normal healthy people because high glucose levels feed the virus and can cause a "cytokine storm" or an out of control immune response. (to learn more see my book The Body Map VI, The Endocrine System - available next year)

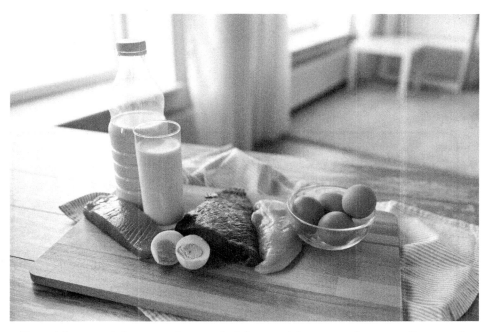

Life Without Diabetes: The Definitive Guide to Understanding and Reversing Type 2 Diabetes - by Roy Taylor, M.D.

For more than four decades, Dr. Roy Taylor has been studying the causes of diabetes. In 2017, he had a breakthrough: he found scientific proof that Type 2 diabetes is not only reversible, but that anyone following a simple regimen can prevent and cure it. Dr. Taylor's research shows that Type 2 diabetes is caused by too much fat in the liver and pancreas, which interferes with both organs' normal functioning. By losing less than 1 gram of fat, the liver and organ can begin to perform as they were designed to once again—thus beginning the reversal process.

- Description from Amazon.com

"For decades we have been taught that fat is bad for us, carbohydrates better, and that the key to a healthy weight is eating less and exercising more. Yet despite this advice, we have seen unprecedented epidemics of obesity and diabetes. The problem lies in refined carbohydrates, like white flour, easily digested starches, and sugars, and that the key to good health is the kind of calories we take in, not the number." - Gary Taubes - *Good Calories, Bad Calories* - Publisher: Knopf;

II

OUR JOURNEY

By Cindy & Tim Cocklin

Cindy: The Journey Begins

We thought it might be a good idea for you, the reader, to know a little about us in order to understand why Tim would consider or have the audacity to write such a technical book when he is not a medical doctor. Our journey begins simply enough for two young people to meet in college, become friends and start to explore the world. We have had the privilege to grow up and old together. I believe God knew we would be a good match, although it would take years to flow in that! Tim's biggest quest in life is to seek truth and understand it. Whether it was the Bible, his career as a system's engineer or how to build a deck, he invariably researches, carefully studies a matter, and finds the best way to move forward. He is constantly looking for something new and a better way to do something. His eye was always on the finish line. Perhaps it wasn't the most elegant analogy, but I use to say; he was the racehorse running towards the finish, and I was the plow horse keeping his furrows straight! We both came from Iowa farms, raised with the Midwest integrity and hard work. Our values, fortunately, were united in our faith in God, America and our future.

However, life has a way of moving forward in ways we don't regularly want. Working, raising children, and being too busy, you don't pay attention to your health in the ways you should. We had little or no health issues when we were young as many do, but slowly things began to creep in and steal our energy.

We had the usual weight gain that many experience when we first married, before the craze of being slim was in vogue, and our first encounter with a 'diet' was the popular Atkins diet at that time. It worked; we felt energized, and the weight loss was fairly quick and easy. We ate the Standard American Diet (SAD) and continued to live our life.

We were transferred to Texas for Tim's career and decided it would be a good time to have another child. Our daughter was born after we had been married two years. I actually got pregnant with her by surprise. I do NOT say by accident after realizing it is not an easy venture to get pregnant. Everything has to be perfectly timed and orchestrated in order for the life to even be created. Something we found to be the case once we decided to have another child. Four years of charts and planning and still no child. Infertility, a more common occurrence now, than 20-some years ago, seemed to be an issue for us. To seek help was expensive and the remedies that are so readily available today were not there at that time. We were willing to surrender to it and be thankful for our beautiful daughter we already had. Finally, I did get pregnant and went for about four months before I miscarried. This began, for me, a roller coaster of health issues of short-term pregnancies and miscarriages, followed by recoveries. My health was affected with all the complications of these female issues, from a cyst on the ovaries, fibrous tumors in the uterus and a slow breakdown of my immune system. We had considered a permanent solution to end the cycle and just give it over to God. I always had a check about walking away and giving up. Please keep in mind, we had no angst regarding the inability to have another child, but I certainly do understand and have tremendous compassion for women who had the same struggles. All around you see women bearing children with no effort and wonder what is going on with you. We were thankful, as I said, for our daughter, and were willing to walk through the other side of this – at peace with what was there. However, God had a different plan. A little more than 13 years after our daughter, I discovered I was pregnant yet again. We had stopped all the attempts and just went about our lives, so this one wasn't exactly planned by us. The only few times I have truly had a Word from the Lord, was this one. I literally heard the Lord speak to my heart- "This one you will bring home." The pregnancy was difficult, with some bumps in the road and a few false alarms, but all ended with the birth of our son.

The years of this, however, broke down my immune system and my health slowly declined. A cold became pneumonia; the flu took weeks to recover, and I suffered constant flu-like symptoms. My body began to break down – the thyroid, the liver, the red blood cells in the bone marrow, and a wide variety of other issues, as well as the ongoing female issues I battled. Until one day, I found myself unable to care for myself and my young son. Tim traveled constantly, and we had no family in Texas to rely on. It was so bad; I was sent to Iowa to live with my sister to help care for us. There were a number of tests that were done with no clear results as to what the cause actually was. I believe it started with an extreme case of chronic fatigue and expanded from there. I realized then that doctors were no different than the rest of us; they were guessing (even though it was an educated guess) as to what was causing the breakdown. Trying unusual remedies, I continued to get worse. I feared that I would not make it to my son's 5th birthday.

[I now believe that she suffered from NAFLD - Non-alcoholic Fatty Liver Disease, we will define that later in the book, but at the time they could not understand why her liver was equivalent to that of an alcoholic even though she did not drink - Tim]

When someone is gravely ill in a family, it affects everyone around them. My daughter, Tim and certainly our young son were all 'damaged' by this event. I say damaged, because at the time it felt like everything was being destroyed. My faith in God and His ability to heal that I had been taught all my adult life came into question. I realize this isn't exactly a biological or physical testimony and what I did to get better. However, you cannot have a true health journey without acknowledging the Creator in all that I experienced. Something unusual occurs when someone is that sick. You are more aware of your surroundings. The more I decided to trust the Lord regardless of the outcome, the more peaceable I became. He actually became more real, more personal and certainly His presence was stronger than I had ever experienced before (and I was one of those 'Jesus freaks' from the 70's!) I began to look at all the different aspects of my life, my family dynamics, my children, our marriage through an unusual perspective. My prayer stopped being "Oh Lord, HEAL ME" and instead became Lord, teach me how to live for you, whether it is for 6 more months or 60 more years." It no longer mattered which it was. There was a magnificent peace and well-being in that. I am not saying I gave up; I had the privilege of going to a marvelous doctor in Iowa- the only one that was taking new patients, would take my health insurance from Texas and happened to be a very strong Christian, who prayed for all his patients. He was definitely God directed, and I am forever grateful to Dr. Benjamin Solomon in Iowa for his dedication to his practice and his patients and more importantly our Lord! He said something very unusually for a doctor. "I am not sure what exactly caused all this breakdown, but you are like a train with all the cars derailed, not just one. It would take too long to try to figure it all out. You won't live long enough. All I can do is fix the things I know to fix and let the Lord guide and direct me, and He will have to fix the rest." And so, it began; it took me a year to recover fully. Not only did I physically get better, but those things that would plague me with worry and anxiety I began to let go. My fears began to be released to the Lord, my desires changed, and I began to see what really mattered, who was important and how much the Lord cared for us all. It was liberating. I came out stronger and more resolved to trust God instead of worry my way to the next event. Little did I know what was ahead for us and how valuable that would be.

Coming back to Texas again was a difficult adjustment just as anything that caused major change to our lives would be. I used to joke that Tim traveled six weeks out of the month. He would normally get home on a Friday night and fly out either on Sunday night or early Monday morning. Training all over the US with a different group in a different city was the variety he loved and embraced the lifestyle. It was a high-stress environment and created his own health issues we didn't see creeping up.

Shortly after I returned in better health, he had an accident, passed-out in a hotel room and injuring himself. He seemed to recover fairly quick, we repaired the broken teeth, and we didn't give much thought as to why he fainted in the first place. A little less than a year later, he began to get headaches, once again; he just credited it to stress and moved forward. I need to explain a little about a few of his strengths. Tim was rarely sick and when he was, he just wanted to be left alone and would sleep it off. He actually has an extremely high pain tolerance, which didn't always work to his benefit. It gave him the ability to push through and basically ignore the pain that a normal person would immediately seek a remedy for. He was not the typical male baby. I had to learn to read him and be sure he took action, which later proved to be an important skill. He was in New Jersey, training, when the headache became so severe he actually asked to be taken to the hospital. Keep in mind that was after he had finished the training for the week! I got a phone call from him- he wasn't sure where he was or what was the issue, just hospitalized. I began to call all the hospitals in the area, and finally found him. He had a brain tumor! I caught the next flight out, and they determined to give him steroids to help 'shrink' the tumor enough and stabilize him in order to have the brain surgery in Dallas, Texas instead of New Jersey. Once home we scheduled the surgery, put him on our prayer list and many people began to pray and intercede for him. NEVER underestimate the power of prayer. One of the prayer partners told us that they thought the Lord would dissolve the tumor. We thought, why not; nothing is too hard for God. When he went to surgery, all they found was a brown liquid, no tumor. The surgeon came out to let me know and wasn't sure how to explain it, mentioning that perhaps the tumor had hemorrhaged and/or moved deeper into the brain, and they were unable to remove it. I laughed and told him the 'Word' we had received. I could tell he perhaps thought of me as one of "those" people and politely said, "Well, that is as good of an explanation as anything else." However, I scheduled a follow-up MRI to ensure we were indeed 'tumor-free'. Six weeks later, the test was absolutely clear and the liquid they kept for diagnosis came back undiagnosable. He was tumor-free and apparently no cancer or anything else.

This was the beginning of Tim's journey. We all have our journey, and sometimes it is difficult and discouraging. However, because of my previous time, the Lord prepared us to walk through this together and come out stronger. There were many events, the company he worked for went bankrupt, and we actually had to reinvent ourselves several times. We had some adventures, lived in an RV with our son, traveled to Florida, participated in the real estate industry and had a few experiences that we would NOT want to go through again, but would not trade for what it brought us in our faith and with each other. Tim was once again traveling and training and began to experience severe, what he thought might be back or shoulder pain, and then it would go away. As usual, he powered through but one night it was pretty severe, even for him, and I took him to the hospital – they couldn't actually see a heart attack and went with the back-pain diagnosis and sent him home. A few days later, it came back, and I once again insisted we have it checked. This time they found some blockage in the heart and put in a stent. His recovery was quick and not much thought was given after that.

We moved back to the Dallas, Texas area and settled in to be near our daughter and grandchildren. Grateful to be back and have all our family in one place and to support our daughter was a wonderful experience. However, Tim began to fail and his energy, vitality and quality of life began to interfere with his daily tasks. Fortunately, he worked from home and could schedule his appointments with clients and still be able to rest during the day. We were on the SAD (Standard American Diet) and thinking we ate fairly healthy, but the weight gain was out of hand, and we knew, for both of us; we couldn't function that heavy. We tried the HGC diet- both lost a lot of weight and felt great. It was also during that time that Tim began to have issues with his blood sugar and was fast becoming a type two diabetic. Not knowing a lot about that, we took the advice and sometimes medicine prescribed by the doctors with little long-term benefits. What we did notice, during the HCG diet, his blood sugar would return to normal and stay that way for a long period of time. We continued to use the HCG program usually a couple of times a year. It would always reset his blood sugar, lose the weight we would gain, but issue was every time we would go on the diet; we would regain the weight and eventually return to the same problems.

During that time period of weight loss, weight gain, and blood sugar up and down, we discovered that the medicines were not doing the job, if anything he was getting worse. He began to experience some severe discomfort and years after the first stint Tim had two heart attacks- 2 weeks apart with 6 stents. The blood sugar, weight and health were slowly getting worse. Everyday was a battle to follow the program given. The statins prescribed for the heart had side effects that were not clearly explained and caused too much fatigue, aches and 'foggy' head that Tim found working difficult.

I was on a constant battle with weight gain and losses that it was extremely discouraging. Every time I would lose 30 or 40 pounds I would gain back that and possibly more. Tim began to study and do his own research to try to find an answer to the issues, the medicines he was taking were not the answer. One drug would do this but cause that, so it felt like a constant battle. We were told that the diabetes would be there for the rest of his life, and he would need to accept that. We couldn't. There had to be a better answer. There are so many resources today that anyone may take charge, ask questions, seek answers for their own health and the lessons we learned years before took effect: be responsible for your personal health. I cannot explain this part of the journey without also saying through much prayer and believing God, who created us, He would have an answer on how to fix us. There are some things that come about by a painstaking walk and experience and others that have happened simply by his mercy and healing. We expected both. Our weight and diet were things we have to walk out and discover what works for our bodies. In the research Tim began to do, he discovered the Keto diet and the effects carbohydrates have on our body, and the damage processed sugars and foods do to us. We noticed that when going on the very restricted HCG diet (no sugars, carbs, etc.) the body responded and his BS would react by being normal. When we returned to the SAD (Standard American Diet) the BS would begin to go up, the weight would come back quickly, and we were unable to maintain the weight and energy we wanted. The problem with that diet is, it only allows 500 calories and tricks your body into burning fat. It does allow you to lose weight quickly, and it is encouraging to get such fast results, but coming off the 500 calories; our metabolism had slowed down, especially for me, that it took little or nothing to gain at least 10 pounds back that I had lost. We needed a way of life, not a diet. One that we could easily live with, get physically fit with and keep for years to come instead of the yo-yo diets of the past.

Whatever we do; we tend to like to do together. It makes it easier, and encourages each other, so we both went on the Keto – very strictly- Tim started to lose weight, actually went from a size 46" waist down to a 38" waist. The digestive issues, bloat, etc. he has always struggled with began to get better. And most of all, his BS was normal without using ANY drugs. So, no side effects plagued him. I would like to say overnight everything was great and healed, but it has been a slow process, experimenting with what his body responds to best and what foods work better.

For me, I struggled with the carb addiction. I always had a desire for bread and sweets, and the first couple of weeks were difficult as I came down from those effects. I noticed a certain freedom when I could go to the store or be at work with 'treats' and not really even desire them anymore. There was more of an emotional attachment to the food versus a physical need for it. It made it easier to ignore the impassioned need for sweets without the constant craving for them. However, the weight loss is still a process for me. I am stuck and do not see the quick results that Tim has seen. They say that may be typical for a male versus female, especially the older you are. I realize our bodies have to repair and heal in order to acquire a health and weight that can be maintained for the rest of our lives.

As I have mentioned before, going through a challenge to your health, finances, or family, isn't just about the one issue. We took these losses and gains, victories and defeats, gave them to the Lord and expected some good to come of it. We, many times had to believe that all things work for good to those who love the Lord. Our job was to learn how to love the Lord and each other through them. Trust me, there were many days we wanted to give up with the problems and each other. When I say that we have had the privilege to grow up and grow old together, it is the thing we are the most grateful for. We married very young and spent all of our adulthood learning how to live and walk a Christian walk through it all. We know how fortunate we have been to preserve over the years.

How difficult it can be when everything you hoped for and planned for doesn't work the way you thought. There will always be more challenges, more difficulties ahead. Tim wrote the book to encourage others to research for your answers, question what is happening and how to make it better and most of all to remind us that God isn't finished yet, so we shouldn't be either.

I want to thank Tim for the opportunity to share a little with everyone who reads this and hope it may encourage you. - **Cindy Cocklin**

Tim: The Journey Continued - A New Lifestyle

I guess you could classify me as a "Johnny come lately" because the information for this book has been available for years, as early as the late 1800s with William Banting and in the 1950s with Dr. Richard Mackarness, with Dr. Atkins in the 80s and recently many others whom I will quote throughout the book. I believe the information has been suppressed by the nutritional establishment (food and drug). I was not aware of this information until 2019! I know that there are likely millions of others have not been acquainted with this information and continue to live without hope. It is for those, like myself who did not know this information that I am putting my story into a written form. If you are or have been diagnosed as a type II diabetic, you are obese, and have other serious illnesses, there may be hope for you even if you have a disease like Multiple Sclerosis or other autoimmune diseases, just ask Dr. Wahls.

> Dr. Terry Wahls MD was diagnosed with progressive Multiple Sclerosis (MS). Dr. Wahls reveals how she recovered her own health and went on to develop a protocol and research to help others heal from autoimmune and chronic conditions. - https://terrywahls.com/

You can find medical professionals who will help you reverse the disease; I pray before there is irreparable damage. I have a growing list of doctors in appendix B, along with other resources that have helped me and others overcome diseases without drugs.

> *Reminder: I am researching the issues; I am not a licensed doctor and do not practice medicine. You need to contact a practitioner who has the right to diagnose and treat your issue, see appendix B for a list of practitioners. Nothing in this book should be taken as medical advice.*

I was diagnosed with type II diabetes. This book is a compilation of the research I have done in order to reverse the disease. After a period of time, the drugs that were prescribed were ineffective. I thought; "**why am I taking all these drugs, which are not solving the problem just prolong it**."

The Band-aid Approach to health

If you pick up a broken drinking glass and get cut, the logical thing to do is put a bandage on the cut to stop the bleeding. But, what if you used that same glass, every day and got cut every day, and you put a bandage on the cut... every day? You do that every day, and every day you put on a bandage. Would you eventually stop to wonder why you are getting cut, and that you need a bandage every day to stop the bleeding? It seems ridiculously simple but the way the medical industry works is to put a bandage on the cut but NEVER take the time to find the underlying cause of the cut. The cure is simple, stop using the broken glass! The medical profession's only concern is to stop the bleeding. Eventually, if you are curious, you would like to know why and what could be done to stop the bleeding every day. You would not just keep putting on a bandage everyday would you? That is what I finally realized about diabetes. I am putting a bandage on everyday, in the form of drugs, and I am not getting better! I had to discover the underlying cause of diabetes. Was there an answer to my problem or do I just go on putting on a bandage every day? I decided to find out what the underlying cause may be and see if it could be addressed and reversed.

I was determined to get off all the drugs which I had been prescribed. **DO NOT** do what I did without a medical professional. I quit taking all the drugs in rebellion this is very unwise in most cases! In some cases, you must be weened off some drugs slowly or suffer dire consequences. I understand now that doctors are taught to prescribe drugs to address health issues. Doctors are trained to address symptoms NOT causes!

They do not have the time to address lifestyle changes to restore health. Since they only get a very small fraction of nutritional training (some doctors have said as a little as four hours) I don't think their nutritional advice carries much weight, and dietitians are indoctrinated to follow the guidelines they have been trained to suggest. Appendix B has a list of dietitians who know the truth and will recommend an alternative. The old-school dietitians will generally suggest a low fat/ low-calorie diet using as their basis the infamous food pyramid and suggest that you exercise more. I suggest they read a book by Denise Minger called *Death By Food Pyramid*. Although, if you follow those who follow their advice, you find a reoccurring theme. "I lose the weight but it comes right back" or for some, the hunger gets the better of them, and they quit. They try the same thing over and over with very poor long-term results. What are they told? "It is your fault you are too lazy, or you didn't follow my advice correctly." Those comments are not helpful. The problem is that their advice, if following the common low/fat eat lots of grains simply does not work long term.

However, there are people I know who would rather take a drug rather than follow a new lifestyle in which they are not accustomed. Sometimes the reversal of maladies like diabetes and obesity can take time. At first, it may be difficult to make the transition to a new lifestyle. Do not give up, stay the course, get sound medical advice from doctors who have a proven track record of addressing your particular issue. There is hope for a better life without disease and pain. Please, get help from a doctor, who has a proven track record of reversing your disease or pain. Appendix B has a list of some who have proven ways to help.

There is additional detail available from the books, videos and website sources I quote in appendix B. You will find a number of competent medical doctors and researchers, which have come to the conclusion that current accepted advice and practices dealing with the issue of physical health are deeply flawed.   If you look at the growing number of people who are obese and burdened with the scourge of diabetes you will have to agree, we have an epidemic of Biblical proportions that is not being addressed appropriately! It is time to stop putting a bandage on everyday. The answer is before us, but it will take time for the change to come because there is so much money involved and those who are profiting from the illnesses will resist the change like drug companies and food manufacturers. Do you remember the cigarette companies that advertised their product as harmless and enjoyable? It took years for the change to take place, and now many have quit smoking. I believe that the recent reduction in heart disease is the result. Billions were spent to promote a lie and millions died as a result. The jury is still out on the consequences of vaping, but putting a man-made chemical in your body will most likely not end well.

Case in Point: Helena, Montana - coincidence or fact?

A smoking ban was implemented June 2002. The heart attack admissions fell during the six months the ban was in force. After the repeal of that ban, admission for heart attacks returned to previous levels. - British Medical Journal - BMJ 2004;328:977

Reduced incidence of admissions for myocardial infarction associated with public smoking ban: before and after study

"Results: During the six months the law was enforced the number of admissions fell significantly (− 16 admissions, 95% confidence interval - 31.7 to - 0.3), from an average of 40 admissions during the same months in the years before and after the law to a total of 24 admissions during the six months the law was effect." - *BMJ*

https://doi.org/10.1136/bmj.38055.715683.55

For some, the change will come too late. I pray that you are not one of those that are too late to get the help you need. There are a number of medical professionals who are joining the cause to stop obesity and diabetes by suggesting the lifestyle I will reveal in this book. I can tell you from personal experience that there is an answer to obesity and the plague of diabetes, and it does not include starving yourself. In appendix B, there is a short list of medical professionals who can help you reach your goals.

I grew up on a farm in Iowa, looking at pictures from back then I was generally thin and healthy. I was never overweight until I got married. I do not blame my wife; she loves to cook and entertain. She likes variety and foods that taste good. It was, however, a change in the diet that resulted in my gaining weight. I have never been one who "lives to eat" if I get hungry I would eat. Nevertheless, being married, I would eat three meals a day hungry or not. Over the years, I would gain weight then lose it repeatedly. My wife and I tried most of the latest craze diets, and chemical concoctions that came along. I ended up with a weight in excess of 285 pounds and was diagnosed with type II diabetes, most likely from the yo-yo dieting followed by diabetic drugs.

The first successful diet I tried was the Atkins' Diet. I had just graduated from college. During my college days, I had the task of unloading 40,000-pound freezer trucks by moving the load on to pallets. With the Atkins diet and a heavy workload, I began to lose all the excess weight.

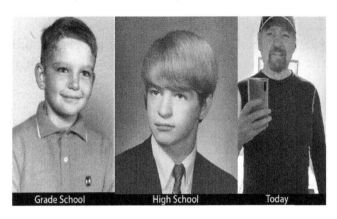

Grade School   High School   Today

I was hired by Texas Instruments before I graduated with a degree in Computer Science. Texas Instruments moved us to Dallas. My job was sedentary. I sat in front of a computer all day. Because we were told that the Atkins diet was detrimental to our health we quit using it. I went back to the Standard American Diet (S.A.D.) and gained all the weight plus a few more pounds. Those I have spoken to who are currently struggling with obesity, diabetes and heart disease have similar stories. The physical labor of unloading trucks may have contributed some to the weight loss, but I believe now the Atkins diet had more to do with it than physical exertion. I do not know who said it but it has been proven to be true: "You cannot out exercise a bad diet". We stopped following the diet based on all the fear mongering about the high fat. The sedentary lifestyle did not help keep the weight off, but it alone is not the reason for weight gain. I found out years later that the "calories in calories out theory of energy conservation" was deeply flawed as I will show throughout this book.

After Texas Instruments, I got a job with a computerized tax preparation company. I was put in charge of the program to direct all the other programs. As a result and an extreme amount of pressure, I worked straight through Thanksgiving day, Christmas day and even New Years day. It had to be done, and it had to work the first week of the year so companies could begin their tax preparation. The extreme stress did cause an increase in my weight.

Later, I was recruited by a Bank Consulting firm in 1984 to create a program to connect the very nascent Personal Computer to an IBM mainframe. I traveled to Los Angeles for over two years on a contract with First Interstate Bank virtually every week. Since we were on an expense account, we ate at the best restaurants in town. My co-workers were used to jogging everyday; I did not join them, so the weight began adding up once again. I have never been a drinker, that was one saving factor and a good thing.

I learned two lessons early in life. First, I learned that gambling does not pay. I was at the State Fair in Iowa, and the Carney kept showing me how I could win a very nice watch. After I lost all my money and had to spend the next few days with no money, I never forgot the lesson. I have been to Las Vegas many times for business, but I have never spent a cent on gambling. Second, when I was a senior in high school, I drank a six-pack of beer. During the next 24 hours, I was so sick; I thought I was going to die. Since that time, I have never drunk like that and have at no time since then been drunk. My attitude is that alcohol's only true purpose is as an antiseptic, otherwise, *for me*, it doesn't taste good; it is expensive, makes you sick, and you end up doing stupid things. Now, I have learned that I don't have to live with obesity or diabetes. I quit listening to the diet "Carnies" that told me I could "win" health by eating a low-fat and low-calorie diet, just exercise more, shut up and take the prescribed medications.

In 1997, I had the job of training sales and technical support people how to use and support a new vehicle based wireless data and cellular phone system. I would travel virtually every week to various locations training the employees. One week I had a very bad headache that would not go away. When I went to the emergency hospital in New York, the doctors did an MRI and told me I had a brain tumor on the pituitary gland and put me on steroids. My wife came to New York to fly back with me so the operation could be done at home in Dallas. When they did the operation, the doctors said that a brownish liquid gushed out but there was nothing to biopsy. It may be the drugs they prescribed, or the continuation of a bad diet; it started me down the path to ill health.

In 2003, we were living in the Orlando, Florida area. I was tasked with

32

training new real estate sales people how to sell new homes and use the company's software program. Once in a while I had extreme debilitating pain in the chest that would come on unexpected. If I sat still for a short while it would go away. Finally, the pain became too intense and my wife demanded that we go to the emergency room. The issue turned out to be a blockage, and I was immediately admitted to surgery, and they put in a stint. At the same time, they told me I had high blood sugar and low blood pressure. After the stint, everything seemed to return to normal.

After a few short years, we moved back to Dallas, Texas. I was told by numerous doctors there: "You have destroyed the pancreas and will live with diabetes from this day forward" and "you will need to take these drugs the rest of your life." That was the response wherever I went. They first put me on Metformin, which had minimal results, then later more and more drugs. I am not a big believer in drugs anyway, and we began looking for an alternative. If I went to the dietitians, the doctors recommended they would have recommended virtually everything that made me diabetic in the first place. I went to a major health site that has recommendations for diabetics. What did they recommend? The infamous food pyramid: Heavy on grains, vegetables, fruits and LOW-FAT dairy and "good" fats (according to them); vegetable oils. That diet may work for people who are healthy, but I was not healthy, this recommendation would exacerbate my illness. No thank you! They vilify: butter, beef, bacon, coconut and palm kernel oils. The promote vegetable oils because they will reduce your cholesterol levels, and they may. However, the problem I have with that is that lowering cholesterol is not the answer! You will discover that cholesterol is NOT the bad guy in our health, it is free radicals, inflammation, oxidized dense lipoproteins, and insulin resistance.

We wanted to find a doctor, who would have a more holistic approach to health. We found a doctor, who was listed as a holistic doctor and a very nice guy. We liked him as a person. However, whenever I went to him for a regular check up, he sat before his computer and went down a checklist and started listing all the drugs I was to take. I thought, "why is he using a computer program to treat the disease, doesn't he know how to get rid of diabetes?" The doctors today are trained that diabetes is a chronic and progressive disease and whomever has it will need to be on drugs the rest of their lives. I am sure the computer program made the work of knowing what to prescribe easier. I always had a suspicion that the program was provided to the medical practitioners by the drug companies to sell more drugs, but I cannot confirm that suspicion.

I was told because you have diabetes, you will also need to take a statin to lower cholesterol, and blood pressure medicine. I told him that I did not have high blood pressure, and the response was "it does not matter, because it will help." The list of drugs seemed to grow every time I saw the doctor. Later because the HbA1c was not improved he said I would need to inject Lantis once a week. I was not getting better! And I was getting more frustrated. It was not the cost of the drugs; those were mostly covered by insurance. I knew there had to be an answer. Why, because I believe that the Creator made our bodies to heal itself, if we allow it time and give it the nutrition it needs. In my experience, drugs can be used to prolong an illness. However, if you have an accident, our emergency care in the U.S. cannot be beat and will likely save your life. Nevertheless, for general health and well being, I am not convinced that current guidelines work very well.

Finally, we found a doctor at a fibromyalgia clinic, who had a different approach. He took several vials of blood. He tested for everything under the sun. His approach was more holistic stating that we needed to understand why I had diabetes. This was the first MD that actually had that approach. Then, he suggested that I lose weight. I was 285 pounds at the time. He put me on an hCG diet (stands for human Chorionic Gonadotropin). This is a hormone active in the placenta after implantation during pregnancy. The idea of the diet is that the hCG hormone would help burn fat by injecting the hGC each day and eating a very restrictive diet of 500 calories a day with zero fat. The basic idea was that hCG will burn existing fat. I still don't know if it was the extreme low calorie intake or the hCG that helped me lose the weight. In any case, the diet helped me lose a massive amount of weight. I was using a drug to lose weight. Then I remembered something Zig Ziglar used to say, "you did not gain weight by taking pills you won't lose weight long term by taking pills." Zig was right, each time the weight came back. Why, because the underlying issue of weight gain was not addressed! Because doctor's practice did not take health insurance, we were eventually forced to find another doctor.

It is my opinion that insurance companies would be better off taking the disease prevention approach to health care; it would be less expensive in the long run. I don't spend any money on drugs; I am drug free! However, if the insurance companies are connected with the drug and food manufacturing companies financially they will not follow good advice. It would be simple; focus on prevention and proven health methods, it will lower costs, and we would all be a lot healthier.

After a period of time on statins and diabetes drugs, I had a chest pain, and after a couple of days once again, my wife demanded that we go to the emergency room. There they confirmed blockage again and immediately took me to the cath lab and checked to see where the blockage was. They put three stents in order to open to the blockage. After two weeks, I was back with chest pain. Again, they put in more stents. I am still not convinced I need all of them. However, I am convinced now that what I was eating exacerbated by all the drugs I was taking actually caused the blockage. I will address later what I found out about cholesterol as evidence for my belief. The cardiologist put me on Plavix, which is prescribed to keep the platelets from sticking together. He also added a statin and blood pressure medicine, beta blockers and recommended a stress test. I was concerned because a good friend had just died from a massive heart attack while taking the stress test. I took the test, and found that there was nothing of a major concern at the time.

Later, we found a practice that would take insurance and had the hCG diet. When I did the blood test, it showed a hemoglobin HbA1c of over 10. This was very alarming to them, and the doctor put me back on Metformin and Lantis immediately. I went on the hCG diet again. I started observing that my fasting blood sugar was steadily going down. I had a thought *"could diabetes be reversed?"* Was it, the hCG or some other reason for the decrease in fasting blood-sugar level? This put me on a quest to find the answer to this question.

After two years of gaining and losing weight on the hCG diet, I was going to have dental surgery. The dentist required that I go back to the cardiologist to get clearance for the procedure, since I would be under anesthetics, they did not want to be liable for any heart issues during the procedure. When I told the cardiologist that I was not taking the statin or the blood pressure medicine, he became belligerent and told me if I did not take the statin I would die. I did not tell him that I had not been taking them for over two years! He once again prescribed all the drugs they were trained to prescribe. I picked up the drugs from the pharmacy, but I never ingested them. Rather than listen to doctors who were trained in medical school by the drug companies, I decided to research the cause of diabetes and to see if it could be reversed. I was now on my way to reversing T2D. Later, we will discuss statins.

To lose weight the advice that is generally given is; eat less and exercise more, all calories are the same, along with other advice, which is even less helpful. I did exercise during this time. The special scale at my doctor's office showed that I had more than enough of the recommended muscle mass but the fat mass was too high. Our weekly schedule was and still is Upper-Body weights using machines, Biceps, Triceps, Shoulders, 155 lbs. to 250 lbs. on Monday and Thursday. Lower Body weights using machines 250 lbs. to 425 lbs, including stomach and back machines, Tuesday and Friday. During the week after 6:00 p.m., my wife and I would do 30 minutes on an elliptical machine four times a week, 2.5 to 3 miles. I did not lose any weight during this time and was severely fatigued every day. The doctor's scale also showed an over abundance of body fat especially visceral fat, the worst kind. Visceral fat is located around vital organs and can build-up in the arteries.

I thought that I had found a doctor who understood diabetes, obesity and the cholesterol myth based on information on a website. I set up an appointment with him, but listening to him, I could tell immediately that he did not understand the latest information on diet and statins. I had a blood test, and as I expected the cholesterol was higher than the guidelines set down by the medical establishment. (I will explain later why that is not a problem). His recommendation? "You need to go on a low-fat diet and start a regiment of statin drugs." I will tell you in the chapter on cholesterol why I did not take his advice based on what I now know about cholesterol, statin drugs and from personal experience.

> *Reminder: I am not a licensed doctor and do not practice medicine. You need to contact a practitioner who has the right to diagnose and treat your issue, see appendix B for a list of practitioners.*

Eating the wrong foods and doing inappropriate exercises can be detrimental and counterproductive. This is why getting the right advice is critical to your health. I have observed many people at the gym who year after year made no visible progress, even when enlisting help from an expensive certified fitness coach. It is obvious that these folks are not getting the help they pay for, if they are trying to lose weight. You will discover that it is not the exercise that will help you lose weight. Exercise is good to maintain a strong body, but it has a very limited benefit for losing the excess fat.

Zig Ziglar used to say, "don't go to a fat doctor if you want to lose weight, they either don't think it is necessary, or they don't know how." Doctors are told that diabetes is a progressive chronic disease and cannot be reversed. That caused me to take a risk, and I decided to stop the drugs, which were not doing the job anyway. I decided to do the research myself a very dangerous approach, I do not recommend it. Find a competent doctor, who can monitor your progress. I was determined to beat diabetes or bust.

I went back on the hCG diet. Keep in mind that I had stopped taking all the recommend diabetic drugs long before. I stopped taking the hCG injections after the 3rd week. Since then I have followed a high-fat (good fats), low-carbohydrate diet, I continue to check the blood-sugar level and chart it on my spreadsheet. On average, the fasting glucose level is between 77 and 97. I will also check it throughout the day to see how foods affect the blood-sugar level. So far, there does not seem to be a spike in the sugar level. However, the experts I will site in this book say that is not the whole story, you need to know the fasting insulin level as well. Additionally, I have lost over 25 pounds already at the time of writing this and continue to lose weight, and my health is improving, all with no drugs. The proof is in the results; the low carb/high (good) fat diet works for me. Since then I have been doing a lot of research and found many doctors who believe as I do; the medical profession, the food companies and the federal government are not dealing with the issue appropriately, as a result people are dying and having limbs cut off needlessly, and the cost is out-of-control!

In 2012 diabetes cost The US $245 Billion a year
2018 Diagnosed diabetes costs in America **$327 Billion per year**

American Diabetes Association

Health is a very complex subject, there are many factors that impact our health. Many studies focus on one small aspect of an issue and therefore, come to incorrect conclusions as to why a population is healthy or unhealthy, I keep hearing; ***"Correlation is not causation!".*** The body is incredibly complex, simple answers are not always appropriate.

God created our bodies to function a certain way. When we violate this system by feeding it the wrong fuel or abusing it in some other ways like environmental chemicals, and inappropriate diet, and man made drugs, then trouble is inevitable.

When doing research for my book series *The Body Map* I came across a few relatively new scientific studies. The first was the effect that certain chemicals have on our endocrine system called endocrine disruptors, the second was epigenetics, which controls the expression of our genes by lifestyle and other environmental factors, third is inflammation and the fourth is the effect that stress and poor sleep have on our health. These factors are not initially obvious upon the surface, but have dramatic effects on your body and quality of life. I will address these issues in another chapter.

The New Life Style

I have adopted a new lifestyle. This lifestyle is very low-carbohydrate high-("good") fat (VLCHF). I am never hungry, and I don't have cravings for junk foods like chips and candy bars because I am virtually satisfied all the time. I find myself going for long periods of time without a need or desire to eat. Now, I am only eating once a day, so I go from the evening meal to the evening meal the next day without hunger. I have to admit that some days I will have a few macadamia, Brazil or pecan nuts for a snack.

You will find when you research the lifestyle that some will suggest intermittent fasting. At first, this does not sound like something that would be very easy to do. However, when you are in ketosis your body uses existing fat to supply its energy needs, intermittent fasting then becomes almost routine without forceful intent on your part. The reason you can go longer on the LCHF verses a high-carbohydrate diet is that the body will burn through carbohydrates very quickly, ask any athlete. If you drained all the blood from your body and analyzed it you would generally find that there is only a little over a teaspoon of sugar in the blood stream at any one time. The carbohydrates (glucose) that don't get used right away get stored as fat (I will show the science behind that statement in another chapter). The data below shows my initial progress when I switched from hCG (500 calories restricted diet, which my wife will tell you I did not follow very strictly) to the new LCHF lifestyle with no restriction of calories. I only eat when I am hungry, which is not very often. Many times I have found myself going for 24 hours without eating, and I am not hungry during the day.

My measurements all over my body went down immediately. It was almost shocking how fast my body reduced from a size 46 to a 38 waist, and I am still reducing.

Before the LCHF lifestyle on hGC.

Date	Weight	Blood Sugar	Week
Sunday, January 13, 2019	246	294	
Monday, January 14, 2019	246	249	1
Tuesday, January 15, 2019	246	219	
Wednesday, January 16, 2019	244.9	219	
Thursday, January 17, 2019	244.9	188	
Friday, January 18, 2019	244.70	188	
Saturday, January 19, 2019	242.50	169	
Sunday, January 20, 2019	243.8	153	
Monday, January 21, 2019	244.9	133	2
Tuesday, January 22, 2019	244.9	141	
Wednesday, January 23, 2019	243.4	130	
Thursday, January 24, 2019	242.9	129	
Friday, January 25, 2019	242.90	133	
Saturday, January 26, 2019	242.10	129	

Started the low carb high fat lifestyle:

Date	Weight	Blood Sugar	Week
Sunday, February 3, 2019	242.1	136	
Monday, February 4, 2019	244	108	4
Tuesday, February 5, 2019	244	104	
Wednesday, February 6, 2019	244.5	104	
Thursday, February 7, 2019	244.1	102	
Friday, February 8, 2019	243.50	90	
Saturday, February 9, 2019	243.20	89	
Sunday, February 10, 2019	243.2	102	
Monday, February 11, 2019 2	43.2	87	
Tuesday, February 12, 2019	243.2	92	
Wednesday, February 13, 2019	243.2	104	
Thursday, February 14, 2019	241.2	90	
Friday, February 15, 2019	243.20	96	
Saturday, February 16, 2019	240.10	95	

At the time I wrote this: **219.0** (and falling) **77 - 97** blood sugar stable all day.

Some may try to say that the LCHF diet is unsafe. Even so, many who came before me can attest to the fact that everything has actually gotten better, and some have been on the lifestyle for 40 years or more. There will always be naysayers that want to rain on your parade for one reason or another. I can tell you it has been a Godsend to me. I look better I feel better, and the diabetes has been reversed with absolutely **NO** drugs.

I recently thought I had found a doctor who was up-to-date with the latest information on diet and cholesterol and went to him for a check up. After listening to him for a short time, I could tell he was not going to help. After I took the blood test, as expected, my cholesterol was above the standard guidelines (a common experience on the keto diet). I knew that would be the case knowing what I had seen from several doctors familiar with the low carb/ high-fat diet. The doctor wanted me to get on a regiment of statins and suggested a low fat/ carbohydrate diet. I hit the ceiling! I knew, based on all the research I have done; this was exactly the opposite of what I needed to do. I had decided not to go back and continue to find a local doctor who is up-to-date and not biased by current dietary guidelines. I am totally convinced that it is NOT cholesterol that is the main factor in diabetes or heart disease.

"In the year 2000, 65% of U.S. adults were overweight and 30% obese. 33% of the U.S. population born after the year 2000 will be diabetic."

Mike Sheridan, *Eat Meat And Stop Jogging: 'Common' Advice On How To Get Fit Is Keeping You Fat And Making You Sick* (p. 13). Lean Living INC.

I watched a video on YouTube called "Fat vs Carbs" made by a journalist in Wales who wanted to test the Low Carb/High Fat diet. It is interesting that without exception, all the naysayers were obese or at least overweight. His personal physician appeared to be morbidly obese. The opposition who recommended the LC/HF diet were all thin and healthy. I don't know if that was by design, or it was just the way it was. I had seen most of the pro-LC/HF proponents before so I knew them to be thin and healthy.

I want to reiterate that there is no "one-size-fits-all" diet. Weston Price investigated the diets of various cultures where the people were separated from modern processed food. Each culture had its own style of nutrition. Some ate mostly meat and saturated fats some ate home-grown foods. All foods were natural and unprocessed. The people, isolated from the modern world, were exceptionally healthy. We will address his findings later.

The people of France eat large amounts of saturated fats; the highly demonized fat, and have a population of only 9% corpulent (fat) citizens. Although there are probably other determining factors, the facts indicate that it is not saturated fat while causing the problem of obesity in America. In this book, we will cite up-to-date research by competent professionals who disagree with the currently recommended food pyramid diet.

Be cautious when accepting the results of nutritional studies because they can be skewed by many factors. The researcher can make a study say what they want it to say by craftily manipulating the findings like Anscel Keys did in the 1950s. Often when these studies say they are low carb/high fat. However, their definition of low carb means 75+ grams a day. A true keto diet is less than 25. Additionally, what needs to be disclosed is who is funding the study and often it is not? For instance, having soda companies fund research on the effects of sugar (and they have funded these studies) turn out to be very biased.

> "There is no association between sugar consumption and obesity" - Richard Adamson Scientist for the **National Soft Drink Association** 3/2003

Do you honestly believe that the enormous amount of sugar and sodium in a soda does not affect obesity? If you do, contact me, I have a bridge I would like to sell you in New York City. Otherwise, read the chapter on sugar to find out why I am confident that sugar is at least partly, if not largely to blame for obesity. The real issue today is that virtually everything has natural or added sugar. The food companies have hidden, in plain sight, sugar under a variety of names. We have been programmed to crave foods sweetened by some type of sugar and those with worthless carbohydrates.

The bottom line is eat "real food". Real food is food which is as close to the way it grows in nature without processing. The truth is; it is the quality of the food we eat that makes the difference. If you drink milk, which has been pasteurized and homogenized, then the real food benefits have been destroyed, especially if the milk is 1, 2% low-fat or skim as we have stated previously. If the meat you eat comes from beef, which has been raised on grass and only grass and not corn and grains you will have a more nutritious meal. Why? Beef cattle raised on grains are generally injected with antibiotics and growth hormones because the feed lots they grow in are teaming with fecal matter. The meat from grain fed beef is higher in omega-6 and lower in omega-3. Your body needs both but over abundance of omega-6 will cause health issues. Although, some of the doctors and keto proponents disagree and say that the hormones do not stay within the meat, this requires more research beyond the scope of this book.

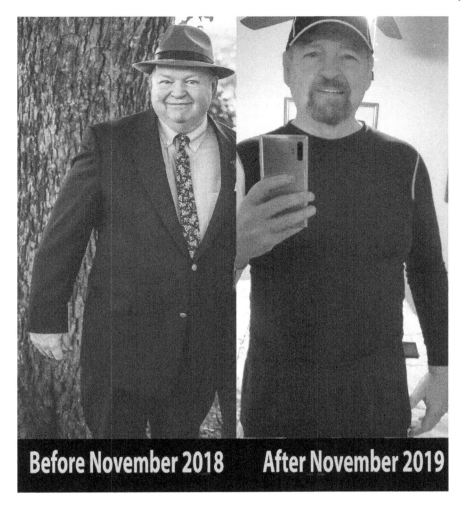

Before November 2018   After November 2019

I was able to reverse type II diabetes within four weeks all without drugs and within 3 months I lost most of the weight. I maintain it even now by eating a Keto/Carnivore diet.

"It is important for Americans to recognize that, despite all of the fancy gimmicks and perceived power of modern medicine, the largest explosion of preventable, chronic diseases ever in the history of mankind has occurred as a direct result of modern medicine and scientific reductionism. Modern medicine is not an antidote for the incredible harms caused by the modern food industry, but it is an effective distraction."

— Charles C Harpe, Naturvore Power

Section 2

What are the Physiological Issues of Diabetes, Obesity & Metabolic Syndrome?

"At the end of our clinic day, we go home thinking,"The clinical improvements are so large and obvious, why don't other doctors understand?" Carbohydrate restriction is easily grasped by patients: Because carbohydrates in the diet raise the blood glucose, and as diabetes is defined by high blood glucose, it makes sense to lower the carbohydrate in the diet. By reducing the carbohydrate in the diet, we have been able to taper patients off as much as 150 units of insulin per day in 8 days, with marked improvement in glycemic control even normalization of glycemic parameters." - Eric Westman, MD, MHS

III

WHAT CAUSES DIABETES, OBESITY AND METABOLIC SYNDROME

I believe based on my interaction with doctors that prevention is not in the vocabulary of most. They are not taught to prevent disease but, only offer treatments after the fact. Additionally, most Americans don't go to a medical professional until they have an issue. It is entirely up to us to live in a way that will promote good health. However, in this book, you will find that the food and drug industries and the so called "health organizations" have lead us astray by giving us bad advice on diet since 1977. This is evidenced by the fact that since the new guidelines were introduced in 1977, the incidence of obesity and metabolic diseases have gone up precipitously!

> **Over 50% in the US have diabetes or are pre-diabetic.**
> JAMA 2015 [The Journal of the American Medical Association]

Diabetes - Disease, virus or what?

"Disease: a disordered or incorrectly functioning organ, part, structure, or system of the body resulting from the effect of genetic or developmental errors, infection, poisons, nutritional deficiency or imbalance, toxicity, or unfavorable environmental factors; illness; sickness; ailment". - Dictionary.com

It came as a surprise to me that diabetes (type II) is not a disease like cancer or a virus like the flu, but it is a food-related syndrome. The doctors told me that diabetes cannot be cured because the pancreas has been irreparably damaged. This may be true for some who have had the issue for decades, even that may or may not be true. And yet, today I check my fasting blood sugar, and it is between 77 to 97 every morning. I am losing weight, and the blood pressure is well within the normal range. I take NO drugs. How did I get here? I want you to understand exactly what diabetes is, it is unlikely that the medical profession will tell you in any detail. The drug and medical industries are interested in treating the symptoms, but not curing or preventing the illness. After much research, I have found a way to reverse the deleterious effect of diabetes. The following is an abstract from a paper explaining the benefits of using a carbohydrate-restricted diet to reverse diabetes:

"Diabetes is the inability to metabolize the load of glucose entering the body" Dr. Gary Fettke

Dietary carbohydrate restriction as the first approach in diabetes management: Critical review and evidence base

The inability of current recommendations to control the epidemic of diabetes, the specific failure of the prevailing low-fat diets to improve obesity, cardiovascular risk, or general health and the persistent reports of some serious side effects of commonly prescribed diabetic medications, in combination with the continued success of low-carbohydrate diets in the treatment of diabetes and metabolic syndrome without significant side effects, point to the need for a reappraisal of dietary guidelines. The benefits of carbohydrate restriction in diabetes are immediate and well documented. Concerns about the efficacy and safety are long term and conjectural rather than data driven. Dietary carbohydrate restriction reliably reduces high blood glucose, does not require weight loss (although is still best for weight loss), and leads to the reduction or elimination of medication. It has never shown side effects comparable with those seen in many drugs. Here we present 12 points of evidence supporting the use of low-carbohydrate diets as the first approach to treating type 2 diabetes and as the most effective adjunct to pharmacology in type 1. They represent the best-documented, least controversial results. The insistence on long-term randomized controlled trials as the only kind of data that will be accepted is without precedent in science. The seriousness of diabetes requires that we evaluate all of the evidence that is available. The 12 points are sufficiently compelling that we feel that the burden of proof rests with those who are opposed.

- The Authors:
Richard D. Feinman Ph.D.a,, Wendy K. Pogozelski Ph.D., Arne Astrup M.D.,Richard K. Bernstein M.D., Eugene J. Fine M.S., M.D.,Eric C. Westman M.D., M.H.S., Anthony Accurso M.D., Lynda Frassetto M.D.,Barbara A. Gower Ph.D., Samy I. McFarlane M.D., Jörgen Vesti Nielsen M.D., Thure Krarup M.D., Laura Saslow Ph.D., Karl S. Roth M.D., Mary C. Vernon M.D.,Jeff S. Volek R.D., Ph.D., Gilbert B. Wilshire M.D., Annika Dahlqvist M.D., Ralf Sundberg M.D., Ph.D., Ann Childers M.D., Katharine Morrison M.R.C.G.P., Anssi H. Manninen M.H.S., Hussain M. Dashti M.D., Ph.D., F.A.C.S., F.I.C.S.,Richard J. Wood Ph.D., Jay Wortman M.D., Nicolai Worm Ph.D.

The paper makes 12 salient points:

1. Carbohydrate restriction has the **greatest effect** on lowering glucose levels.

2. Caloric increases are mainly due to increased carbohydrates

3. Benefits of low carb do not require weight loss

4. No diet is better than carbohydrate restriction for weight loss

5. Low carbohydrate diets for type II diabetics is frequently better than others

6. Replacing carbohydrates with protein is generally beneficial

7. Dietary total and saturated fat do not correlate with risk for cardiovascular disease (CVD)

8. Saturated fatty acids in the blood are controlled by dietary carbohydrate more than by lipids in the diet (dietary SFA does not correlate with CVD.)

9. The best predictor of micro vascular complications is glycemic control

10. Carbohydrate-restriction is most effective in reducing serum triglycerides and increasing HDL (high density lipoprotein)

11. Carbohydrate-restricted diets reduce and frequently eliminate medication.

12. Intensive glucose lowering by dietary carbohydrate-restriction has no side effects comparable to the effects of intensive drug treatment

"Replacement of carbohydrate with fat or, in some cases, with protein, is beneficial in both types of diabetes leading to better glycemic control, weight loss, cardiovascular risk markers, and reduction in medication. This is what we know. That is what is established in well-controlled experiments in individuals with diabetes (points 1, 3, and 10)."

Dead Food

The food companies, in order to make food taste better, add sugar in various forms and process the food so it can stay on the grocery shelf for an extended period of time. If it is liquid, they will strip all the fiber out, then pasteurize it to keep any bacteria from forming. If a food can set in your refrigerator or on the shelf for an extended period of time, it has been totally processed and is basically dead food. When it comes to bread, first they strip all the nutrients and the fiber out of the wheat.

This will allow it to stay on the shelf or at home for some period of time. Then to make it sound nutritional, they add back nutrients. They call it "fortified with vitamins and minerals." What are these nutrients they are adding? Do these fortified ingredients add or subtract from the real value of the original food? What is the real nutritional value of these man-made concoctions? The more a food is processed, the less real value it has to our bodies. Your body knows the difference! As the commercial used to say "You can't fool mother nature".

They will also change or add things to make the food product more appealing. Some still use MSG (Mono sodium glutamate). This additive, for instance, has severe side effects for some people. These side-effects include; increased blood pressure, Asthma attacks, headaches and other symptoms. You will find that most of the added sugar today is in the form of high-fructose corn syrup, a cheap sweetener.

High-Fructose Corn Syrup (HFCS) is 50% glucose and 50% fructose (NIH The National Institutes of Health). HFCS must be processed by the liver and will be converted to fat or glycogen before the body can use it for fuel. When an excess amount of fructose is consumed it is stored as fat. According to a study by the NIH showed that glucose promoted satiety and fructose did not, leading to a desire to eat more. Later, we will discuss the hormones (leptin and ghrelin) that tell the body that it is full or not.

Effects of fructose vs glucose on regional cerebral blood flow in brain regions involved with appetite and reward pathways. - Page KA1, Chan O, Arora J, Belfort-Deaguiar R, Dzuira J, Roehmholdt B, Cline GW, Naik S, Sinha R, Constable RT, Sherwin RS.

Abstract IMPORTANCE:
"Increases in fructose consumption have paralleled the increasing prevalence of obesity, and high-fructose diets are thought to promote weight gain and insulin resistance. Fructose ingestion produces smaller increases in circulating satiety hormones compared with glucose ingestion, and central administration of fructose provokes feeding in rodents, whereas centrally administered glucose promotes satiety."

Next time you are in the store, check to the label to see how much added sugar there is in the packaged food, being careful because it can be labeled with different names. An excess intake of HFCS is understood to be the major cause of insulin resistance (type 2 diabetes), inflammation and most metabolic syndromes like heart disease, and some cancers. Gout is often associated with the consumption of meat. However, sugar also increases the levels of uric acid (hyperuricemia).

See the table for a partial list of sugars found in our food.

The following is a partial list of sugars you may encounter in your food:		
		blackstrap
agave nectar	barley malt	molasses
brown rice syrup	brown sugar	coconut
sugar		
cane sugar	corn syrup	date sugar
dextrin	diastatic malt	dextrose
ethyl maltol	Florida crystals	fructose
fruit juice	glucose	golden syrup
high-fructose corn syrup	honey	lactose
levulose	maltodextrin	muscovado
maltose	maple sugar	molasses
nonfat dry milk	palm sugar	panocha
sorgum syrup	sorbitol	saccharose
skimmed milk	powder sorghum	sucrose
treacle	turbinado	

Thanks to Louis Pasteur we have a process known as pasteurization. Pasteurization is the process of heating the liquid up to a kill all the bacteria. Unfortunately, that process destroys most of the nutritional value of the liquid but the liquid will have a much longer shelf life.

We are told that high blood sugar is the result of the pancreas not making enough insulin to keep up with the amount of sugar flooding the blood. The first question that must be asked, but is often not, why is there excess sugar in the first place?

All carbohydrates turn into glucose. When the cells of our body become saturated with glucose the cells effectively close the gate that accepts it. Where does this excess glucose go? In the case of a diabetic, it floats around in the blood or it is stored as fat.

Diabetes Type II

It is my opinion that type II diabetes can be reversed. Type I, however, is a result of a pancreas incapable of secreting insulin at all when sugars get too high and therefore must inject insulin to remain healthy. In this book we will only concern ourselves with type II.

According to the Centers for Disease Control and Prevention. National Diabetes Statistics Report, 2017. Atlanta, GA: Centers for Disease Control and Prevention, U.S. Dept of Health and Human Services; 2017. (CDC) 30.3 million people have diabetes (9.4% of the U.S. population) Those who have been diagnosed: 23.1 million people. Those who are undiagnosed 7.2 million (23.8% of people with diabetes are undiagnosed).

Diabetes is a non-communicable disease where the cells in the body can no longer take in sugar (insulin resistance) and therefore, leaves the excess in the blood stream. Some of the initial symptoms are; frequent urination, increased thirst and often increased hunger. Left untreated this situation can cause complications, which are very severe and sometimes deadly. Many type II diabetics have to get limbs cut off as a result of high blood sugar. Other problems associated with type II are; nerve damage, dental disease, eye issues, kidney disease, strokes and heart disease. It is my opinion that it does not have to be this way.

According to a video presentation by Dr. Robert Lustig of the University of California average per total global population figures:

(Visit: http://www.uctv.tv)

Calories Consumed per day		% with Diabetes
1985: 2655 calories		1985: 0.62%
2010: 2866 calories		2010: 5.13%
an 8% increase in calories	BUT	**727% increase in diabetes!**

World Sugar Consumption

1985: 98 million tons   2010: 160 million tons

Global Diabetes Prevalence

1985: 30 million people   2010: 346 million people

What we can learn from Dr. Lustig's figures? It is not calories, but the type of calorie that is being consumed that causes the problem!

The World Health Organization (WHO) estimates that by 2030 there will be **552 million** with diabetes!

What causes a normally health person to be overcome with type II diabetes?

1. Insulin Resistance

The pancreas sends insulin into the blood stream. The insulin unlocks the cells receptor allowing the cell to take in sugar (glucose). Insulin is an anabolism for storing glucose in the cell which can be used to generate energy in the Mitochondria. Insulin is a fat storing hormone produced in the pancreas by the beta cells. Studies have shown that adding insulin will actually cause you to gain fat! Dr. Jason Fung proclaims he can make anyone fat by giving them insulin. Over time if the diet creates an excess amount of sugar and fat the cells of the body get "full" they become resistant to the effect of insulin. At some point the pancreas cannot produce enough insulin to keep the blood sugar from getting too high, because the cells reject it.

Insulin resistance does not always mean that the pancreas is not pumping out enough insulin but the cells have gotten to the point they can not accept more sugar. Some drugs attempt to force the cells to accept the excess sugar. Dr. Jason Fung compares that procedure to the Japanese subway system where people are hired to shove people in the train after it is full.

Lipogenesis (the process of turning glucose into fat) occurs when insulin levels get high. The opposite is also true, when insulin levels are low, fat can be removed. This is why some drugs, which keep insulin levels high, will not allow a person to lose weight! It also can cause weight gain.

Type II Diabetes does not come on quickly but builds up over time as the body becomes more and more insulin resistant. Eating the Standard American Diet (S.A.D.) with a lot of simple carbohydrates; breads, pastas, starches, and sugars over time can lead to diabetes. Other contributing factors include: stress and issues with sleep. I can say from personal experience that when I cut out sugar, simple carbohydrates and high-glycemic foods, that my blood sugar normalized and I began to lose weight!

When insulin levels are high, several detrimental things happen in the body: weight gain, an increase in visceral fat (around vital organs), hypertension (high blood pressure), inflammation in several parts of the body, and the mitochondria (the cell's energy source) start to malfunction among other issues. This is the result of high-carbohydrate intake.

2. Obesity, Overly Processed Food and Sugar

Why do people get obese? Is it because these people are lazy, undisciplined? That may or may not be true, however, I do not believe that to be true for most people. There are genetic issues that may come into play for some. If you ask virtually any doctor or dietitian how to lose weight, they will tell you to go on a low-calorie/low fat diet and exercise more. We have stated before that scenario only works in the short run and is normally always followed by increased weight gain and reduced metabolism. The answer is in what people eat, we will discus that later.

According to data from the National Health and Nutrition Examination Survey (NHANES), 2013–2014

More than 1 in 3 adults were considered to be overweight.
More than 2 in 3 adults were considered to be overweight or obese.
More than 1 in 3 adults were considered to have obesity.
About 1 in 13 adults were considered to have extreme obesity.
About 1 in 6 children ages 2 to 19 were considered to have obesity

You can see from graph #1, on the next page, that obesity and extreme obesity have increased dramatically since the 1960s by following the advice of the "experts" and eating a diet of low-fat/ low calorie in various forms. We have already illustrated what has happened since the "experts" made their recommendations in the 1970s:

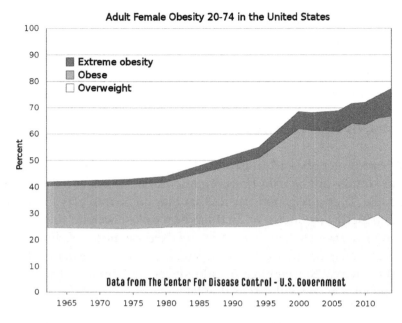

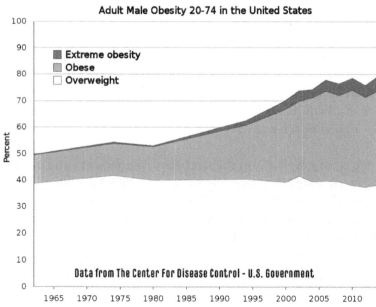

Graph #1

What the "experts" told us is that saturated fats from meats, butter and cholesterol from eggs cause heart disease. They tell us that fat from these sources will make you fat. Their recommendations include vegetable oils and low-fat sources. Then came the low-fat craze everywhere we saw an increase in low-fat foods. Even today we see foods in the store which tout reduced or low-fat. The issue with these low-fat foods is when you remove the fat, you remove the flavor. In order to make the low-fat food palatable they must add sweeteners. You can see from the table below that since 1980s chronic diseases have advanced rapidly!

From an Article · May 2016 Richard Lear - Brown University

The Root Cause in the dramatic rise of Chronic Disease
See discussions, stats, and author profiles for this publication at:
https://www.researchgate.net/publication/303673576

Autism (2,094%)	*Alzheimer's* (299%)
COPD (148%)	**diabetes (305%)**
Sleep apnea (430%)	celiac disease (1,111%)
ADHD (819%)	asthma (142%)
Depression (280%)	*youth bipolar disease* (10,833%)
Osteoarthritis (449%)	lupus (787%)
Inflammatory bowel (120%)	chronic fatigue (11,027%)
fibromyalgia (7,727%)	multiple sclerosis (117%)
hypothyroidism (702%)."	

The chapter called Sugar - Pure, White and Deadly will explain why this is a very bad idea. I challenge you to look at the label of food that is said to be good for you. If it claims to be low-fat, what percentage of the food is carbohydrate and what percentage is sugar. The food companies are very adept at hiding sugars by using other names. (see the table on sugar names on a previous page.) In some cases they get away with saying they are sugar free. That is only technically true, nevertheless, it is a deception.

Some people have a high metabolism and can eat virtually anything and not gain weight, others are not so blessed. The food today is overly processed removing all the natural nutrition and adding back fillers, man made vitamin concoctions, sugars and carbohydrates. Many restaurants have exchanged good fats for highly processed "vegetable oils". We will discuss the dangers of these processed fats and sugars in another chapter.

There is one proven way to reverse type II diabetes. I do not recommend this method because of the adverse effects it can and will produce: Gastric Bypass surgery. This method re-routes part of your digestive system so you don't absorb as much food. There are many issues with this procedure; vitamin and mineral deficiencies, weakness, sweating, fainting, gallstones, nausea, and reflux. There is a better way and it is dietary, drug free and requires not surgery.

Diabetes is often associated with obesity, however, there are people who are obese who are not diabetic and there are people who are not obese that are diabetic. The underlying issue of diabetes is insulin resistance.

THYROID HORMONES

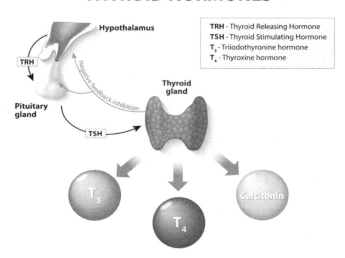

Causes of Weight Gain

Under-active thyroid gland (hypothyroidism) - This is a case where the thyroid does not produce enough of the hormone thyroxine (also called T4). Symptoms of hypothyroidism are: tiredness, weight gain, depression muscle aches, dry skin and temperature sensitivity.

The hypothalamus sends a message via the Thyroid Releasing Hormone (TRH) to the pituitary gland. The pituitary produces thyroid-stimulating hormone (TSH) which directs the thyroid gland to produce its hormones.

An iodine deficiency can be linked to hypothyroidism. Iodine is a mineral that is used in the production of thyroid hormones. If iodine is not sufficient then the thyroid hormones can not be created effectively. There are nine minerals that are required for the thyroid to complete its tasks: iodine, selenium, zinc, molybdenum, boron, copper, chromium, manganese, and magnesium.

The thyroid hormones triiodothyronine (T3) and thyroxine (T4), can change the way the body processes fat.

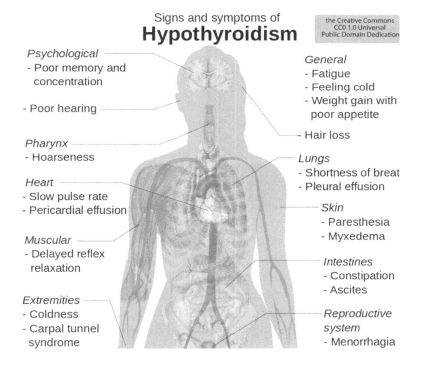

Signs and symptoms of
Hypothyroidism
the Creative Commons
CC0 1.0 Universal
Public Domain Dedication

Psychological
- Poor memory and concentration

- Poor hearing

Pharynx
- Hoarseness

Heart
- Slow pulse rate
- Pericardial effusion

Muscular
- Delayed reflex relaxation

Extremities
- Coldness
- Carpal tunnel syndrome

General
- Fatigue
- Feeling cold
- Weight gain with poor appetite

- Hair loss

Lungs
- Shortness of breat
- Pleural effusion

Skin
- Paresthesia
- Myxedema

Intestines
- Constipation
- Ascites

Reproductive system
- Menorrhagia

T4 is converted to T3 in the organs and tissue. T3 the active form of thyroid also influences the regulation of metabolism. Once the body has reached homeostasis the thyroid sends negative feedback to the hypothalamus to stop sending TRH to the pituitary.

RT3 or reverse T3 is created in the body to rid the body of any excess T4. The liver is a chief creator of RT3. Cirrhosis of the liver can be the cause of increased RT3. Diabetes that is not under control can also increase RT3. There are other reasons as well. An increase in T3 will increase hypothyroidism.

Metabolic Syndrome - (75% of all healthcare dollars are spent here)

Metabolic Syndrome is defined by having at least 3 of the following disorders: high blood sugar, high blood pressure, excess fat around the midsection (see below), high blood triglycerides and low high-density lipoprotein (HDL), Non-alcoholic fatty liver disease, Polycystic ovarian disease, cancer, dementia.

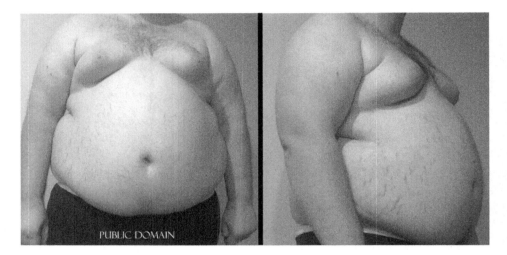

PUBLIC DOMAIN

Contributing factors to metabolic syndrome: chronically high insulin levels and inflammation. Why does your body increase the insulin levels? By having a chronic overabundant amount of glucose in your blood brought on by excess sugar intake or carbohydrates which turn into glucose, to the point where the cells become insulin resistant. High levels of insulin will keep the fat cells from releasing fat to be used for energy.

Inflammation on the other hand is often associated with eating toxic foods like "vegetable oils". They should be called seed oils because these oils are made from seeds like cotton seed, soybeans and corn, safflower, sunflower. The process needed to make these oils is frightening. It is a process using high heat, petroleum products, chemicals to change the color to a more appealing tint and a process to remove the offensive smell. See the chart to see how "Vegetable Oil" is made.

Making Vegetable oil

Canola, Soybean, Corn,
Sunflower, Safflower
(not vegetables but seeds)

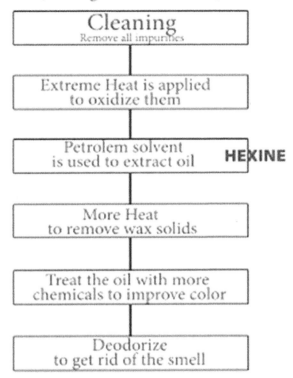

Cleaning
Remove all impurities

Extreme Heat is applied
to oxidize them

Petrolem solvent
is used to extract oil **HEXINE**

More Heat
to remove wax solids

Treat the oil with more
chemicals to improve color

Deodorize
to get rid of the smell

These polyunsatured fats (**PUFAs**)
are unstable These fats are easily oxidized
and therfore cause inflammation and
mutation of cells. The Vegetable (seed) oils
are high in Omega 6

To make margarine
Hydrogenate until solid

"Saturated fat and cholesterol in the diet are not the cause of coronary heart disease. That myth is the greatest scientific deception of this century, perhaps any century."

– George V Mann M.D. Co-Director of the Framingham Study

Dr. Jason Fung makes a statement that he could make you fat by injecting insulin. Why? Because Insulin is a fat storage hormone.

"More than any other hormone, insulin is the hormone of storage. Think about the function of eating food associated with fuel. Once the "gasoline" (sugar, fat, and protein) is poured into our body as we eat, the body must decide: Burn it or store it?

If insulin is around, the decision is made: STORE IT.

So anything that stimulates insulin production, pushes what you eat into storage. This has implications regarding the main nutritional emergency of our era, obesity. Insulin is a key player in this epidemic.

Clearly eating too much is the true heart of the obesity epidemic. But WHAT you eat, can have a tremendous impact on whether insulin is pumped into circulation and forces what you eat into storage.

Sugar is the top stimulation for insulin production. Eat a bunch of celery and not much insulin will gush to store fuel, but eat a bag of candy and insulin will indeed gush forth, pushing that candy into glycogen in your liver and fat into your fat.

This is a quick path to obesity."

– Dr. Arhur Lavin,
   Food: How Fats, Sugars, and Proteins Go to Work

"The simplest way to look at all these associations, between obesity, heart disease, type 2 diabetes, metabolic syndrome, cancer, and Alzheimer's (not to mention the other the conditions that also associate with obesity and diabetes, such as gout, asthma, and fatty liver disease), is that what makes us fat - the quality and quantity of carbohydrates we consume - also makes us sick."

— Gary Taubes, *Why We Get Fat: And What to Do About It*

"An obese person... may be given a diet of meat, excluding bread and potatoes, and the patient will reduce to his normal weight. As soon as the patient returns to his diet of bread and potatoes, he begins to increase in weight".

— Dr. Emmet Denmore (1892) from his book: **How Nature Cures:** *Comprising a New System of Hygiene; Also the Natural Food of Man; a Statement of the Principal Arguments Against the Use of Bread, ... Pulses, Potatoes, and All Other Starch Foods*

IV

How the Body Works

The human body was designed to operate under somewhat narrow tolerances. If you treat it right, give it the right fuel, the right amount of rest, avoiding harmful environments and as little stress as possible things will go well. If you find utopia where everything is perfect, let me know.

The question is: how does the body work when it comes to fat, type II diabetes and cholestrol?

Adipose Cells (fat cells)

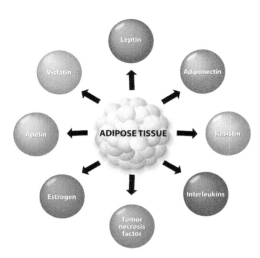

Excess Fat, for some is very difficult to release. You may think, as I did, that fat cells are blobs that just sit there and accumulate fat, not true. What do adipose cells actually do? Fat tissue is beneficial for storing energy, insulation, cushioning. In terms of endocrine functions adipose cells will produce Leptin, Adiponectin, resistin, angiotensinogen and cytokines.

Leptin signals the hypothalamus and gives you that sensation of being full so you will stop eating (satiety). Conversely, the hormone Ghrelin, produced from the cells of the stomach, signal the hypothalamus that you are hungry. Unfortunately, individuals with Prader-Willi syndrome will have increased Ghrelin levels and will therefore be hungry most of the time and will have a propensity to over eat making them obese.

> Prader-Willi syndrome is caused by the loss of function of genes in a particular region of chromosome 15. People normally inherit one copy of this chromosome from each parent. Some genes are turned on (active) only the copy that is inherited from a person's father (the paternal copy) is on. This parent-specific gene activation is caused by a phenomenon called genomic imprinting.
>
> https://ghr.nlm.nih.gov/condition/prader-willi-syndrome#genes
> (see also *The Body Map - Reproduction*)

There are those who have a leptin insensitivity and never fill satisfied. In either case the individual becomes obese.

igure 4. Trends in age-adjusted obesity and severe obesity prevalence among adults aged 20 and over: United States, 999–2000 through 2017–2018

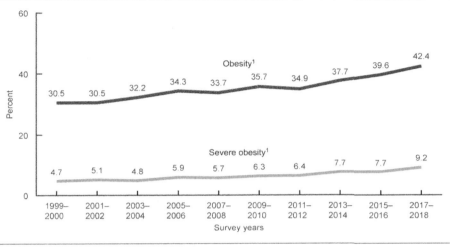

ignificant linear trend.
OTES: Estimates were age adjusted by the direct method to the 2000 U.S. Census population using the age groups 20–39, 40–59, and 60 and over. Access da
ble for Figure 4 at: https://www.cdc.gov/nchs/data/databriefs/db360_tables-508.pdf#4.
OURCE: NCHS, National Health and Nutrition Examination Survey, 1999–2018.

SOURCE: NCHS, National Health and Nutrition Examination Survey, 2017–2018

How did I get fat in the first place?
[This is an over simplification of the process but illustrates the point]

It starts when eat. The intestines extract the nutrients from the food. Then chylomicrons (ultra low density lipoproteins) are created which package triglycerides, phospholipids, cholesterol, and proteins to be delivered to the cells. Since the fats and cholestrol are oily and the blood is watery, the contents have to be encased in the lipoprotein (chylomicrons) so it can be delivered to the cells through the blood.

The pancreas puts insulin in the blood stream to open the cell to accept the glucose. The body cannot store unlimited amounts of glucose. When the cells have been saturated the cells turn off the insulin receptors and will not accept more. At this point the excess must go somewhere. This excess ends up in body fat.

The enzyme Hormone-Sensitive Lipase (HSL) when active will break down fat in the adipose cell and release it for energy. However, HSL is the inverse of insulin which stores fat. If you are eating an excess of carbohydrates which are not used for energy, then insulin will increase and HSL will decrease causing the storage of fat in the adipose tissue.

Things that may help:

1. Lower you intake of carbohydrates, causing **insulin levels to fall**.
2. Intermittent fasting, causing **HSL to increase** (more on that later)
3. high-intensity interval training causing EPOC (Excess Post-exercise Oxygen Consumption).

Do you ever get hungry during the day and eating a candy bar, chips or fruit makes that hunger disappear? Your body is telling you that it has run out of glucose and wants more. This is a vicious circle because glucose is used up quickly and you will find that you need an "energy" boost again. This endless cycle will cause you to store fat. This means that you will not be able to use existing stored fat because insulin levels have risen.

Why can't I lose weight?

We have said that the recommended way to lose weight most often suggested is: "eat less and exercise more". I would guess that if you have been trying to lose weight you have tried that method, I know I have. But, it did not work for me and I would guess it did not work for you. Do not get me wrong, exercise is good, however, we in the USA exercise more than any other country but are still the most obese. What exercise is best? The experts I have learned from say; high-intensity interval training (HIIT). This type of exercise involves quick, intense burst of exercise that raises your heart rate. Intervals are typically a 1:2 ratio. Example: one minute of intense exercise followed by a two minute rest.

Calorie restriction will work initially but your metabolism will decrease so in order to lose more weight you must taken in even less calories. I know I have tried that and I would guess you did as well. Unfortunately, this cycle of less and less calorie intake results in abandoning the idea altogether because it cannot be maintained, but now, because your metabolism is lower, when you go back to eating normally you will gain all the weight you lost and will generally gain even more weight. The HCG diet we tried did help us to quickly lose weight but it all came back with a vengeance!

High intensity training in obesity: a Meta-analysis
Y. Türk,corresponding author W. Theel, M. J. Kasteleyn, F. M. E. Franssen, P. S. Hiemstra, A. Rudolphus, C. Taube, and G. J. Braunstahl
Published online 2017 May 29. doi: 10.1002/osp4.109 PMCID: PMC5598019

Objective
to determine the effectiveness of HIT on cardiopulmonary fitness and body composition in adults with obesity compared to traditional (high volume continuous) exercise.

Conclusion
Training at high intensity is superior to improve cardiopulmonary fitness and to reduce %body fat in adults with obesity compared to traditional exercise. Future studies are needed to design specific HIT programs for the obese with regard to optimal effect and long-term adherence.

The Danger of a low calorie diet is the shortage of glycogen. If there is not enough fuel, the body will then take muscle tissue and break it down as a sugar through a process of gluconeogenesis. In a sense the body is in the process of cannibalizing itself. This generally explains why you can lose muscle mass while on this type of diet even if exercising vigorously. The other issue is that your metabolism is reduced meaning that to lose additional weight you must consume fewer calories. At some point the dieter is frustrated and gives up, it is a vicious cycle.

The absolute worst thing you can do is go on a plan then off and then back on again. This "yo-yo" dieting will result in havoc with your metabolism. I have heard of people who try the low-carb life style for a while and then because of a birthday, a holiday or celebration will go off and go back to the S.A.D. diet. When they return to the LCHF lifestyle they have difficulty losing weight. When I first started on the very low carbohydrate, high good fat life style, I had what is known as the keto flu as I switched from carbohydrates for fuel to fat for fuel. It manifests itself very much like the flu. That was short-lived and I have not had that feeling since then. At the time of this writing I have not had a cold, or flu for over 2 years, not even a sniffle. Headaches are virtually nonexistent. I cannot guarantee you will have the same result, but I was obese and had type II diabetes, both are gone.

You may have had the belief that eating fat will cause you to gain fat. That is about as far from the truth as you can get. However, not all fats are equal. If eating a low fat diet worked we would all be thin. Go down any isle in the store and you will find a multitude of products touting that they are low fat and heart healthy. We have learned that food companies can pay to use the "Heart Healthy" label so be careful when choosing food that has that designation. Remember we are in an age of mis-information, please check out for yourself what anyone says, especially the "experts".

> *Reminder: I am researching the issues; I am not a licensed doctor and do not practice medicine. You need to contact a practitioner who has the right to diagnose and treat your issue, see appendix B for a list of practitioners. Nothing in this book should be taken as medical advice.*

The Types of fat

Considered by some nutritionists as <u>bad fats</u>:
(*actually they are* not bad, these will help you lose fat)

Saturated: Dairy, unless you are allergic to dairy (whole: milk, butter, ghee, cheese and cream), eggs, coconut oil and meats

Mono-saturated: Olive Oil (cold pressed), Lard

Considered by some nutritionists as <u>good fats</u>:
(*Chemically these* are bad we will explain why)

Polyunsaturated Fats: Corn Oil, Cotton Seed Oil, Soybean Oil, Safflower Oil, Peanut Oil, Canola Oil

Trans fats: Hydrogenated oils - according to the Mayo Clinic trans-fat is the worst type of fat.

Considered by all as <u>good fats:</u>
Omega 3s: Fish Oils, Flaxseed

The Omega fats:

Omega 3 - polyunsaturated fat (essential the body can not make them)
    anti-inflammatory
Omega 6 - polyunsaturated fat (essential the body can not make them)
Omega 7 - Palmitoleic Acid - monounsaturated fat
Omega 9 - Oleic Acid - monounsaturated fat

Vegetable ("seed") oils
https://www.youtube.com/watch?v=7kGnfXXIKZM

Dr. Chris Kobbe gave a very interesting talk at the Low Carb Down Under in Denver Colorado, June 13, 2020. He gives a time line of processed foods:

- 1822 to 2009 sugar consumption increases 17 fold
- 1866 Cotton Seed Oil was introduced
- 1880 refined wheat flour came on the scene
- 1911 P&G introduce Crisco (trans fats)
- by 2009 63% of the American diet is processed food (USDA)

"Vitamins A, D, and K2 and not found in vegetable sources not even in good oils like avocado, coconut or olive". These come from meat and egg sources.

Use of PUFAs went from 0 grams of the daily diet in 1880 to 80 grams in 2010. Dr. Kobbe points out that one third of our diet comes from seed oils. In 1900 99% of fats came from animal fats by 2005 86% of fats came from vegetable oils.

Dr. Kobbe illustrates that the three extremely healthy populations; the Maasai in Africa, the Tokelau Islanders of the Pacific, and the Tukisenta of Papua New Guinea have this in common: no refined sugar, no refined wheat, no processed foods, no vegetable oils. He contends that it is not carbohydrates that are harmful 17% in Maasai and 95% in Tukisenta. It is not the fat content 2.4% in Tukisenta and 66% in the Maasai. He goes on to illustrate the types of fat are not the problem either the saturated or the monounsaturated.
Dr. Kobbe explains that the excess omega-6 in our diet causes a reactions in the body which are very destructive. The issues in oxidative stress and inflammation. The end result is mitochondrial dysfunction and a cascade of ill effects occur: insulin resistance, neuro degeneration (Alzheimer's, Parkinson's), Cancer, obesity and heart failure.

Sugar burning vs Fat burning

If you are not losing weight (fat), the issue most likely is that you are not burning fat but sugar. In order for food companies to make their product taste good after removing the fat, they add sugar in some form. This puts you in an never-ending cycle of burning sugar and not fat. Carbohydrates are burned first before stored fat. At some point if you have ingested excess carbohydrates, the body cannot burn it for fuel and begins to store it. Then to make matters worse, if the cells are saturated, they will begin to reject more sugar, then the pancreas will start pumping out more insulin to force the excess into the cells. When the cells refuse to take it, the excess goes into the blood stream this then if not corrected can lead to a diabetic state. If not corrected can end up causing a plethora of problems from mild to death threating. This is what is happening in the country right now and why we see a dramatic increase in a multitude of diseases. In the case of a type II diabetic the body becomes insulin resistant, therefore, increasing the amount of insulin in the body is ineffective! It is the same with leptin, (the hormone that tells you that you have eaten enough) feeding your body more of the hormone leptin does not work because the hypothalamus becomes insensitive to it. Then you have the issue inflammation caused by sugar, grains, toxins and bad fats as stated above.

How do I lose weight then?

It is a matter of what you eat plus the hormones; leptin, HSL and insulin (and many more beyond the scope of this book). As an adult, the amount of perceived fat in your body is due to the size of the adipocyte (fat) cell. When you lose size, you are actually reducing the size of the adipose cell. [Liposuction attempts to remove adipocyte cells from the body. However, the result is short-lived since the issue of fat storage has not been addressed]. The fat is stored as a triglyceride. Triglycerides are too large to be transported into the cell directly; an enzyme is required to break it down. Insulin increases the response to the stimulus of the enzyme

lipoprotein lipase. The enzyme will break down the fat into free fatty acids. The result of this process will allow it to be transported into the cells. The effect of Insulin will move the GLUT4 transport (a protein) to the surface of the cell bring the glucose in to be used by the cell. There are many other factors going on here, but to make it simple, Insulin regulates in flux and out flux of fat and glucose (sugars). Too much insulin will cause fat to be stored; lower levels of insulin will cause fat to be released for other purposes other than storage.

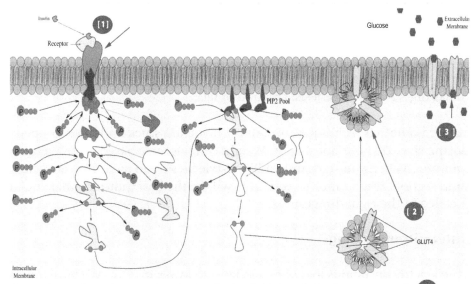

The insulin signal transduction pathway begins when insulin binds to the insulin receptor proteins [1] Once the transduction pathway is completed, the GLUT-4 storage vesicles [2] becomes one with the cellular membrane. As a result, the GLUT-4 protein channels become embedded into the membrane, allowing glucose to be transported into the cell [3]

Wikipedia contributors, "GLUT4," Wikipedia, The Free Encyclopedia, https://en.wikipedia.org/w/index.php?title=GLUT4&oldid=951675638 (accessed June 10, 2020

It is said that carbohydrates are necessary because they feed the brain and the energy it needs. Not true, there is an alternative source; Keytones.

How do you get into a fat-burning mode? You fix hormone resistance and inflammation by lowering the amount carbohydrates you ingest. In 1898, Dr. Richard Williamson in his book *Diabetes Mellitus and Its Treatment* said, "Potatoes should be excluded from the diet first, then bread, and gradually all carbohydrates should be cut off." He did not know what we know today so I assume his recommendations were based on experience. Almost one hundred years earlier in 1797 a military surgeon John Rollo M.D. in his book *An Account of Two Cases of the Diabetes Mellitus* suggested a high fat, low-carbohydrate diet. Captain Meredith, one of his patients, lost a great deal of weight and the diabetic symptoms were reversed. I can attest that this way of eating works, without drugs and without hunger.

Since the body will burn carbohydrates first, if you flood the body with carbohydrates and the resulting sugar is not used at the time, insulin levels rise and the process starts that results in fat being stored in your adipose cells. When insulin levels rise the hormone leptin often does not get activated so you don't get that "feeling" of being full and cycle continues and if not checked problems begin to rise. The excess glycogen, is created in the liver through a process known as de novo lipogenesis. (de novo: Latin meaning new & lipogenesis: creation of fat).

There is another technique you can try if you are stuck and have stopped losing size. Yes, size not weight. Weight can fluctuate based on the retention of water. When you start an LCHF lifestyle be sure to measure your chest, mid section, thighs and the rest. This will be the best indicator that you are headed in the right direction.

Intermittent fasting.

The key to continuous loss of excess fat is to lower insulin. We have touted the idea of eating fat. However, fat can still raise insulin levels. OK, I have reduced carbohydrates and increased my ketogenic lifestyle, but I am not getting anywhere. The next step would be intermittent fasting. There are many benefits to fasting.

Believe it or not fasting causes growth hormone to increase and HSL as mentioned before. The result is you start burning fat to preserve lean muscle tissue and adrenaline kicks in giving you more energy. When you fast you burn the available glucose, this puts you into ketosis where you start to burn fat for fuel instead of glucose. Studies have proven that intermittent fasting lowers insulin and leptin resistance and increases HSL.

Because the body is in a constant state of flux, you can accumulate damage to your cells, and waste can increase. This accumulation can interfere with normal cellular functions. Intermittent fasting can kick off a process known as autophagy. Autophagy is the "cleaning lady" of the body because it sweeps the body of toxic proteins and promotes the regeneration of health cells. Autophagy may even help reduce neurodegenerative diseases like Parkinson's and Alzheimer's, reduce inflammation and enhance the immune system.

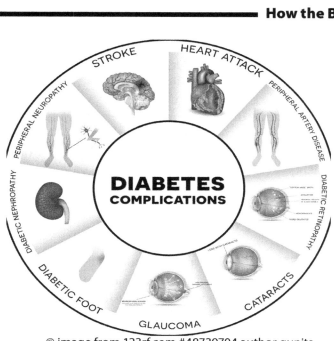

© image from 123rf.com #48739704 author gunita

There are many ways of intermittent fasting,

- 5:2: eat normally for five days and two days only eat 600 calories.
- O.M.A.D. eating only once a day fasting the rest of the day. (this is what we normally do)
- 16:8: eat within a short period of time (8 hrs) in any 24-hour period

The idea is to let your body catch up and start the autophagy process (see the chapter on hidden factors). I have found that if I am eating a sufficient amount of good fats, that I am not hungry so intermittent fasting becomes easy.

> "Instead of using medicine, better fast today" - Plutarch (45AD - 120AD)

The question you may have at this point is: is the ketogenic safe or will it have long lasting ill effects? We turn to a study of 83 obese patients for the answer.

Long-Term Effects of a Ketogenic Diet in Obese Patients
https://www.ncbi.nlm.nih.gov/pmc/articles/PMC2716748/pdf/ecc09200.pdf

OBJECTIVE: To determine the effects of a 24-week ketogenic diet (consisting of 30 g carbohydrate, 1 g/kg body weight protein, 20% saturated fat, and 80% polyunsaturated and monounsaturated fat) in obese patients.

(Personally I would have used a higher percentage of saturated fat and no polyunsaturated fat but even with bad fats the results were good...)

PATIENTS AND METHODS: In the present study, 83 obese patients (39 men and 44 women) with a body mass index greater than 35 kg/m2 (77.16 lbs), and high glucose and cholesterol levels were selected. The body weight, body mass index, total cholesterol, low density lipoprotein (LDL) cholesterol, high density lipoprotein (HDL) cholesterol,

triglycerides, fasting blood sugar, urea and creatinine levels were determined before and after the administration of the ketogenic diet. Changes in these parameters were monitored after eight, 16 and 24 weeks of treatment.

RESULTS: The weight and body mass index of the patients decreased significantly (P<0.0001). The level of total cholesterol decreased from week 1 to week 24. HDL cholesterol levels significantly increased, whereas LDL cholesterol levels significantly decreased after treatment. The level of triglycerides decreased significantly following 24 weeks of treatment. The level of blood glucose significantly decreased. The changes in the level of urea and creatinine were not statistically significant.

CONCLUSIONS: The present study shows **the beneficial effects of a long-term ketogenic diet. It significantly reduced the body weight and body mass index of the patients. Furthermore, it decreased the level of triglycerides, LDL cholesterol and blood glucose, and increased the level of HDL cholesterol.** Administering a ketogenic diet for a relatively longer period of time did not produce any significant side effects in the patients. Therefore, the present study confirms that it is safe to use a ketogenic diet for a longer period of time than previously demonstrated.

Type II diabetes

Diabetes is a very serious condition where too much sugar is left in the blood stream. Over 90% of diabetes is type II. Increased levels of insulin can weight gain and other serious issues. If not corrected, you can see in the illustration in the previous page that many complications can result.

Are you diabetic? You could be if you have these symptoms:
- Increased thirst
- Increased urination
- Blurred vision
- and many other symptoms.

What causes Diabetes Type II?

Dr. Gay Fettke says "*diabetes is the inability to metabolize the load of glucose entering the body*". If you overload the system with sugar producing foods at some point the human system cannot keep up by burning the excess. First insulin goes causing the cells to taken in as much as they can. However, at some point the cells become insulin resistant and reject the continual bombardment leaving the sugar in the blood, causing the problems seen on the previous page. Continuing to overload the system with sugar producing foods can eventually lead to a diabetic state. Because the diabetic state is caused by the foods we consume, the foods you choose can also reverse the diabetic state and reduce your insulin resistance.

We have the mistaken idea that sugar comes only from things that are sweet; fruits, candy, and other things. However, Dr. David Unwin has created a chart of sugar equivalence. You may be surprised to learn how much sugar is in different "harmless" foods. A boiled white potato has the equivalent of 9.1 teaspoons of sugar, baked french fries has 7.5, Basmati rice has 10.1. These foods will spike your blood sugar levels. However, foods containing good fats will generally not raise blood sugar, to any great degree. Protein, however, can spike insulin which if overeaten can be harmful, but to a much lesser degree.

NAFLD

Other harmful effects of and overload of sugar or fructose is what happens to the liver. Nonalcoholic fatty liver disease (NAFLD) is the result of a build up of fat in the liver. This problem is closely associated with type 2 diabetes, obesity and metabolic syndrome. The Center for Disease Control estimates that one in five adults have NAFLD and one in ten adolescences. The JAMA (Journal of the American Medical Association), in a randomized clinical trial of 40 adolescent boys with Fatty Liver Disease over an eight week period, found that a diet of low free sugars resulted in a reduction of hepatic steatosis from 25% to 17%. [ClinicalTrials.gov Identifier: NCT02513121]

The New York Times said in an article titled *To Fight Fatty Liver, Avoid Sugary Foods and Drinks* - January 22, 2019 by Anahad O'Connor said "They also had a 40 percent drop in their levels of alanine aminotransferase, or ALT, a liver enzyme that rises when liver cells are damaged or inflamed. "..."As a practicing hepatologist, I see children weekly with fatty liver, and I would love to see this kind of improvement in my patients," said Dr. Vos. "The exciting part was not only did the fat go down, but their liver enzymes also improved. That suggests that they also got a reduction in inflammation."

So, excess sugar is as Dr. Lustig says "toxic" and you find the ill effect of it in many different areas of our health.

Diabetes is it Progressive?

It is said that type II diabetes is a chronic, progressive disease that cannot be cured. *That is true if you only treat the symptoms and do not address the cause.* I can personally attest to the fact that it can be reversed without the use of debilitating drugs. More on this later.

What about the Cholestrol issue?

You will find that cholestrol is not the villain that it is made out to be. In fact studies have shown that the older a person is, the more cholestrol they need. All the drugs that attempt to lower cholestrol do more harm, in many cases, than good. We will explore the statin drugs which attempt to lover cholestrol later.

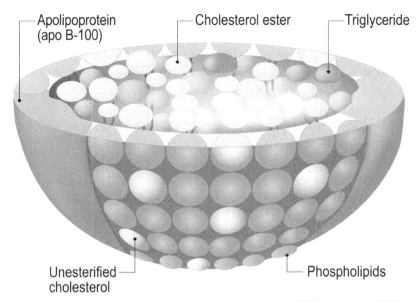

Apolipoprotein (apo B-100) Cholesterol ester Triglyceride

Unesterified cholesterol Phospholipids

https://www.123rf.com/stock-photo/lipid_proteins.html?sti=o81q04d68r2pp3bh09|&mediapopup=97351152

Basically, cholestrol is not **cause** of the arteries getting clogged. Cholestrol appears in a clog as a repair mechanism, to demonized cholestrol is similar to blaming the firefighter for the fire. Cholestrol is critical in so many ways:

- it is found in every cell membrane
- it is found in the brain (25%)
- it is the basis for many hormones
- it helps made bile (necessary to break down fats
- it also helps make vitamin D

The body makes cholestrol, only 25% come from the diet. When you eat, the intestines package **chylomicrons** (Ultra Low Density LipoProtein ULDL) in a protective coating so it can be transported through the blood to feed the cells of the body. Since the blood is "watery" and the fats are "oily", the fat must be packaged otherwise you have and oil and water situation and the content could not be delivered. These chylomicrons are then recycled by the liver. When you are between meals the lipoproteins (containing fat triglycerides, cholestrol and other substances) start out as VLDL in the liver and the transporter drops of its cargo as it travels through the body ending up as LDL (the so called bad cholestrol, and it is not bad at this point). Then the liver recycles the LDL buy reloading content. HDL comes in to play as a mechanism to absorb excess cholestrol back to the liver. LDLs have more than the job of delivering energy to the cells, it will also clear the causes of disease (pathogens) and neutralize free radicals, because they carry vitamin E as an antioxidant. However, if the LDL is attacked by free radicals it changes the chemistry and the receptors on the liver cannot recognize the modified LDL and rejects it. That LDL then floats in the blood stream and can cause major issues.

The LDL particles are surrounded by Apolipoprotein B (ApoB) which cells recognize and will then allow the content into the cell. It is also recognized by liver receptors which then take the LDL out of the blood stream. When you eat a lot of "vegetable oils" like Canola, Corn, Cottonseed, Soy, Sunflower, Safflower, Rice bran, Grapeseed the LDL will appear lower because they are oxidized and will not be counted in your LDL blood work. It appears to help lower your LDL but in fact you get a lot of

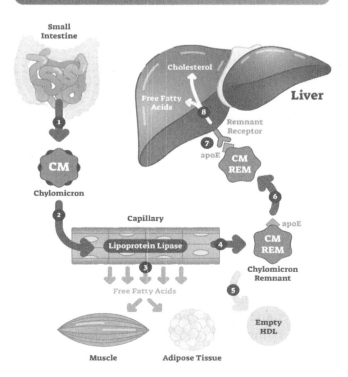

damaged LDLs... NOT good. This process causes a fatty streak the first stage of Atherosclerosis. The white blood cells see the damaged LDL cells as invaders and begin to clean it up. If there is to much damage the white blood cells can not clean it all up so, it can weaken the arterial wall. When the artery wall is breached then the clotting factors come in to do their job and platelets form around the damage.

Cholesterol and All-Cause Mortality in Elderly People From the Honolulu Heart Program: A Cohort Study

I J Schatz 1 , K Masaki, K Yano, R Chen, B L Rodriguez, J D Curb

PMID: 11502313 DOI: 10.1016/S0140-6736(01)05553-2

Background: A generally held belief is that cholesterol concentrations should be kept low to lessen the risk of cardiovascular disease. However, studies of the relation between serum cholesterol and all-cause mortality in elderly people have shown contrasting results. To investigate these discrepancies, we did a longitudinal assessment of changes in both lipid and serum cholesterol concentrations over 20 years, and compared them with mortality.

Interpretation: We have been unable to explain our results. **These data cast doubt on the scientific justification for lowering cholesterol** to very low concentrations (<4.65 mmol/L) in elderly people.

Low Cholesterol is Associated With Mortality From Stroke, Heart Disease, and Cancer: The Jichi Medical School Cohort Study

Naoki Nago,1 Shizukiyo Ishikawa,2 Tadao Goto,3 and Kazunori Kayaba4

Background
We investigated the relationship between low cholesterol and mortality and examined whether that relationship differs with respect to cause of death.

Conclusions
Low cholesterol was related to high mortality even after excluding deaths due to liver disease from the analysis. **High cholesterol was not a risk factor for mortality.**

* Underlining for emphasis

Coronary artery disease and haemostatic variables in heterozygous familial hypercholesterolemia.

D D Sugrue, I Trayner, G R Thompson, V J Vere, J Dimeson, Y Stirling, and T W Meade   PMCID: PMC481754   PMID: 3970784

Abstract
Haemostatic variables were measured in 61 patients with heterozygous familial hypercholesterolemia, 32 of whom had evidence of coronary heart disease. Age adjusted mean concentrations of plasma fibrinogen and factor VIII were significantly higher in these patients than in the 29 patients without coronary heart disease, but there were no significant differences in serum lipid concentrations between the two groups. Comparisons in 30 patients taking and not taking lipid lowering drugs showed lower values for low density lipoprotein cholesterol, high density lipoprotein cholesterol and antithrombin III, and a higher high density lipoprotein ratio while receiving treatment. The results suggest that hypercoagulability may play a role in the pathogenesis of coronary heart disease in patients with familial hypercholesterolemia.

Definitions:
Haemostatic - the process of stopping blood flow.
Heterozygous - dissimilar pairs of genes for any hereditary characteristic.
                    - Dictionary . com
Hypercholesterolemia - higher levels of cholestrol than normal
Plasma fibrinogen and factor VIII - clotting factors
Hypercoagulability - abnormally high coagulability of blood

see my book *The Body Map - Designed from the Beginning* for a more detailed explanation of blood clotting.

According to a presentation by David Diamond *"Demoniztion and deception of Cholestrol Research"* platelet activation and not cholestrol causally linked to risk for CVD (Cardiovascular disease). He sites four factors that contribute: Smoking, Diabetes, obesity, and metabolic syndrome. He goes on the explain how drug companies deceive by using faulty statics. "using statins to lower blood cholestrol is equivalent to bloodletting, taking out a vital substance from the body with drugs".

STAGES OF ATHEROSCLEROSIS

123rf.com: Image ID: 71809948

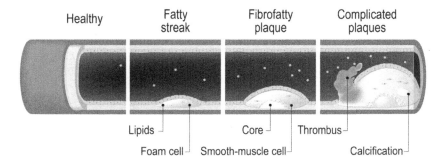

| Healthy | Fatty streak | Fibrofatty plaque | Complicated plaques |

Lipids — Core — Thrombus—

Foam cell— Smooth-muscle cell— Calcification—

> "High LDL cholestrol (LDL-C) and particle count (LDL-P) on a LCHF diet can be a reflection of higher VLDL secretion and use to meet energy demands."— Dave Feldman
> https://cholesterolcode.com

Does eating meat cause gout?

Uric Acid crystals that form in the joins, typically in the big toe, and cause excruciating pain. The first place that people blame is meat, although meat may play a part it is not the cause. Once again we find the firemen are getting blamed for fire simply for being at the fire. Red meat does not cause gout by itself! Research has shown that insulin resistance, fructose and alcohol are most likely the cause. People who quit eating meat and still get bouts of gout should look at their diet. Is the diet filled with carbohydrates? Carbs quickly turn into sugar in the body. Check the label to see how much sugar or fructose is in the product you are about to eat , typically high fructose corn syrup is a main ingredient because it is so cheap to make.

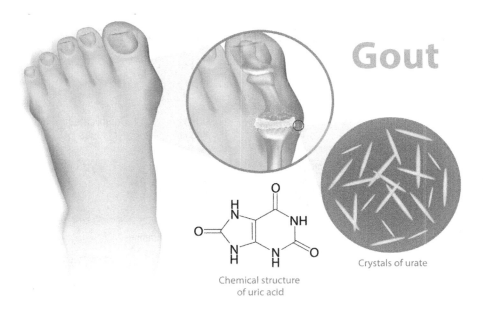

Chemical structure
of uric acid

Crystals of urate

Gout

The people I know who get bouts of gout do not drink alcohol so that would not be a contributing factor.

According to Dr. Paul Saladino two thirds of the uric acid is created in the body itself. That means that only one third comes from your diet. The uric acid comes from the breakdown of purines, ATP to ADP to AMP to IMP (Inosine monophosphate synthase) which is where uric acid comes from when created in the body. The one third comes from purines in the diet. The kidneys are responsible for eliminating excess uric acid. When you are insulin resistant the kidneys do not excrete the excess uric acid. We have addressed insulin resistance in the book, it is an issue when there is an overwhelming amount of carbohydrates in addition to an inflammatory condition. Dr. Saladino blames the over consumption of oxidized omega 6 "vegetable" oils that tend to have worse levels of insulin resistance. So, what he is saying is higher level of insulin means lower levels of uric acid elimination, more uric acid in the blood and a very high change of uric acid crystals being formed in the joints.

High Fructose Corn Syrup (HFCS) was introduced in the US in 1975. We now find HFCS in almost everything! In 1982 the USDA, American Medical Association and America Heart Association suggest lowering fat consumption to stop heart disease. How did that work out? NOT GOOD! According to Dr. Robert Lustig, in 1970 LDL was discovered, They observed that dietary fat caused LDL levels to rise. Therefore because LDL was correlated with Cardiovascular Disease then fat must be the cause of heart attacks. WRONG!

Dr. Lustig lists several things that happen with fructose consumption:

- Forms Advanced Glycation End-Products (AGEs)
- Does not suppress the ghrelin hormone telling you, you are hungry
- Does not stimulate Leptin telling you are full, so you eat more
- Metabolism in the liver is different than sucrose.
- Promotes Metabolic Syndrome.

Regulation of Uric Acid Metabolism and Excretion

Abstract: Overproduction of uric acid, generated from the metabolism of purines, has been proven to play emerging roles in human disease. In fact the increase of serum uric acid is inversely associated with disease severity and especially with cardiovascular disease states. This review describes the enzymatic pathways involved in the degradation of purines, getting into their structure and biochemistry until the uric acid formation.

Maiuolo J, Oppedisano F, Gratteri S, Muscoli C, Mollace V. Regulation of uric acid metabolism and excretion. Int J Cardiol. 2016;213:8-14. doi:10.1016/j.ijcard.2015.08.109

"Our bodies are a complex machine. It is important while you begin the Keto adventure that you stay in touch with how your body works. You may need to research your insulin in the blood, your ketosis level, too much protein or potential issues with certain foods. This may seem complicated at first, but it is vital to be in tune with your health. Don't allow someone or something else decide for you based on "studies" that don't work for you. Take the time, take charge of your own road to recovery. Be accountable for your own future and good health"

. — Cindy Cocklin

And by all means get help if you need it from qualified professionals. I have a short list in appendix B.

Fructose Intake and Risk of Gout and Hyperuricemia: A Systematic Review and Meta-Analysis of Prospective Cohort Studies

Conclusions: Fructose consumption was associated with an increased risk of developing gout in predominantly white health professionals. More prospective studies are necessary to understand better the role of fructose and its food sources in the development of gout and hyperuricemia.

Jamnik J, Rehman S, Blanco Mejia S, et al. Fructose intake and risk of gout and hyperuricemia: a systematic review and meta-analysis of prospective cohort studies. BMJ Open. 2016;6(10):e013191. Published 2016 Oct 3. doi:10.1136/bmjopen-2016-013191 Protocol registration number: NCT01608620.

Quotes from:
https://www.dietdoctor.com/video/mini-documentaries/reversing-type-2-diabetes

Dr. Sarah Hallberg: Diabetes is a chronic disease and it's going to continue to get worse if you follow the guidelines, the guidelines sadly put out by associations that are supposed to be advocates for people with diabetes. So if we want to solve the problem, we have to take away the cause.

Dr. Jason Fung: If you're a type 2 diabetic, it's a dietary disease, it's a disease of essentially too much sugar. So if you understand it like that, then the answer is to get that sugar out, get it down.

Dr. Bret Scher: People with type 2 diabetes should have hope that this is absolutely a reversible condition. If you're following the right nutritional and lifestyle advice and you're getting appropriate support and guidance as you go, yes, you absolutely can reverse this disease.

Dr. Jeffry Gerber: All these diseases in modern society that we treat today we refer to them as chronic diseases ultimately caused by these federal guidelines and unfortunately these guidelines are causing the diseases that we were trying to prevent in the first place.

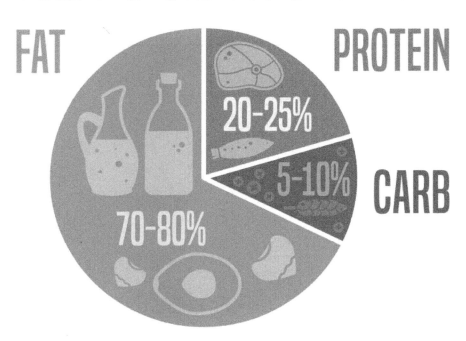

image from 123fr.com Image ID: 111436067

Nevertheless, there is little doubt that small disturbances in endocrine function, particularly during certain highly sensitive stages of the life cycle (e.g., development, pregnancy, lactation) can lead to profound and lasting effects.
Kavlock et al., 1996. EPA, 1997

IV

Hidden Factors that affect your body:

Endrocrine Disruptors, Epigenetics, Inflammation, and more

Endrocrine Disruptors (EDCs)

There are environment issues which do affect the body these are known as endocrine disruptors. Are food and chemical companies knowingly or unknowingly making you fat and diabetic?

A new study by the Endocrine Society says: yes. In the meeting of the International Conference on Chemicals Management (ICCM4), in Geneva, Switzerland, the Endocrine Society stressed the importance of reducing EDCs (the endocrine-disrupting chemicals) found in our food.

Hormones are important in maintaining good health. EDCs work by interfering with the body's natural hormones and therefore, disrupt the ways cells develop and grow. One of the more well known EDCs is bisphenol A (BPA). This chemical is commonly found in plastics, cosmetics; food can linings and many other common everyday products. According to the society, virtually everyone on earth has most likely been exposed to some degree.

About 35 percent of American adults are obese, and more than 29 million Americans have diabetes, according to the Society's Endocrine Facts and Figures report (these facts may be out-of-date are likely higher now).

"Hundreds of studies are pointing to the same conclusion, whether they are long-term epidemiological studies in human, basic research in animals and cells, or research into groups of people with known occupational exposure to specific chemicals."

- Andrea C. Gore, Professor and Vacek Chair of Pharmacology at the University of Texas at Austin - [http://medicalxpress.com/news/2015-09-chemical-exposure-linked-diabetes-obesity.html]

In the article, *Environmental Obesogens: Organotins and Endocrine Disruption via Nuclear Receptor Signaling* by Felix Grun and Bruce Blumberg Department of Developmental and Cell Biology, University of California, Irvine, they state that an increase in calorie intake and a lack of physical exercise contribute to the problem of obesity and diabetes but these may not be the only reasons.

"However, recent findings highlight the possible involvement of environmental obesogens, xenobiotic chemicals that can disrupt the normal developmental and homeostatic controls over adipogenesis and energy balance. Environmental estrogens, i.e. chemicals with estrogenic potential, have been reported to perturb adipogenic mechanisms using in vitro model systems, but other classes of endocrine-disrupting chemicals are now coming under scrutiny as well." - ibid

What they are conveying is that obesogens (chemicals that alter lipid homeostasis and fat storage), can disrupt energy balance or modify the regulation of appetite to promote fat accumulation and therefore obesity. The xenobiotic chemicals, those that are not normally found in our foods, like drugs and chemicals found in our food and environment, will disrupt the normal homeostatic control over the fat cells and energy balance. Some chemicals have an estrogen potential, (usually a woman's hormone) that interferes with normal storage and energy in the cell. Now, they are looking at EDCs as potential progenitors of obesity and onset diabetes.

Their study also indicates that the child is more likely to be obese if the mother is a smoker before or during pregnancy but not necessarily after the birth of the child. Leaving us to assume that chemicals from smoking cross the placenta barrier and affect the development of the child.

Studies have shown that there are at least 20 obesogens commonly found in our environment. The most widely used obesogens are: BPAs, phthalates and perfluorooctanoic acid (PFOA) and to a lesser degree tributyrin.

"Tributyltin is a known obesogen, or chemical that stimulates the development of fat cells — known as adipocytes — and fat storage," said Blumberg. "About 50 chemical obesogens have been identified." Blumberg showed that animals exposed to an obesogen in the womb gained more weight. - Bruce Blumberg, Ph.D., from the University of California, Irvine - from the NIH website.

EDCs fool the body into over responding to stimulus by imitating hormones like insulin when it is not needed. Insulin has been proven to be a fat storing hormone. The EDC can also cause an overproduction or and underproduction of hormones like an overactive or under active thyroid causing weight gain or loss.

> Nevertheless, there is little doubt that small disturbances in endocrine function, particularly during certain highly sensitive stages of the life cycle (e.g., development, pregnancy, lactation) can lead to profound and lasting effects (Kavlock et al., 1996. EPA, 1997).

Bisphenol S is an analog of bisphenol A. It is commonly found in thermal receipts, plastics, and household dust. Traces of BPS have also been found in personal care products.[1] It is more presently being used because of the ban of BPA. BPS is used in place of BPA in "BPA free" items. However, BPS has been shown to be as much of an endocrine disruptor as BPA.[2]
- Wikipedia contributors. "Endocrine disruptor." Wikipedia, The Free Encyclopedia. Wikipedia, The Free Encyclopedia, 17 Jun. 2019. Web. 26 Jul. 2019

[1]. Rochester JR, Bolden AL (July 2015). "Bisphenol S and F: A Systematic Review and Comparison of the Hormonal Activity of Bisphenol A Substitutes". Environmental Health Perspectives. 123 (7): 643–50. doi:10.1289/ehp.1408989. PMC 4492270. PMID 25775505.

[2]. Eladak S; et al. (2015). "A new chapter in the bisphenol A story: bisphenol S and bisphenol F are not safe alternatives to this compound". Fertil Steril. 103 (1): 11–21. doi:10.1016/j.fertnstert.2014.11.005. PMID 25475787.

Endocrine disruptors can:
From: https://www.niehs.nih.gov/health/topics/agents/endocrine/index.cfm

- Mimic or partly mimic naturally occurring hormones in the body like estrogens (the female sex hormone), androgens (the male sex hormone), and thyroid hormones, potentially producing over stimulation.

- Bind to a receptor within a cell and block the endogenous hormone from binding. The normal signal then fails to occur and the body

• fails to respond properly. Examples of chemicals that block or antagonize hormones are anti-estrogens and anti-androgens.

• Interfere or block the way natural hormones or their receptors are made or controlled, for example, by altering their metabolism in the liver.

Abstract - Endocrine-Disrupting Chemicals: An Endocrine Society Scientific Statement
- https://www.ncbi.nlm.nih.gov/pmc/articles/PMC2726844/

There is growing interest in the possible health threat posed by endocrine-disrupting chemicals (EDCs), which are substances in our environment, food, and consumer products that interfere with hormone biosynthesis, metabolism, or action resulting in a deviation from normal homeostatic control or reproduction. In this first Scientific Statement of The Endocrine Society, we present the evidence that endocrine disruptors have effects on male and female reproduction, breast development and cancer, prostate cancer, neuroendocrinology, thyroid, metabolism and obesity, and cardiovascular endocrinology. Results from animal models, human clinical observations, and epidemiological studies converge to implicate EDCs as a significant concern to public health. The mechanisms of EDCs involve divergent pathways including (but not limited to) estrogenic, antiandrogenic, thyroid, peroxisome proliferator-activated receptor γ, retinoid, and actions through other nuclear receptors; steroidogenic enzymes; neurotransmitter receptors and systems; and many other pathways that are highly conserved in wildlife and humans, and which can be modeled in laboratory in vitro and in vivo models. Furthermore, EDCs represent a broad class of molecules such as organochlorinated pesticides and industrial chemicals, plastics and plasticizers, fuels, and many other chemicals that are present in the environment or are in widespread use. We make a number of recommendations to increase understanding of effects of EDCs, including enhancing increased basic and clinical research, invoking the precautionary principle, and advocating involvement of individual and scientific society stakeholders in communicating and implementing changes in public policy and awareness.

- Diamanti-Kandarakis E, Bourguignon JP, Giudice LC, et al. Endocrine-disrupting chemicals: an Endocrine Society scientific statement. Endocr Rev. 2009;30(4):293–342. doi:10.1210/er.2009-0002

Our Understanding of Endocrine-Disrupting Chemicals

"The evidence for adverse reproductive outcomes (infertility, cancers, malformations) from exposure to endocrine-disrupting chemicals is strong, and there is mounting evidence for effects on other endocrine systems, including thyroid, neuroendocrine, obesity and metabolism, and insulin and glucose homeostasis."

"Effects of endocrine-disrupting chemicals may be transmitted to further generations through germ-line epigenetic modifications or from continued exposure of offspring to the environmental insult."

The Endocrine Society Research 2009
https://www.endocrine.org/topics/edc/what-edcs-are/history-of-edcs

One excuse or diagnosis that is often used is: "you are preprogrammed to have the [fill in the blank] because of your genetics!" Statistics disagree; many fatal diseases were not prevalent in our recent past, and your genes do not change that quickly but your epigenetic markers can. My grandmother and her mother did not have diabetes, but my mother did. My siblings do not have it. However, can genetics play a role? Yes, I am not saying there is no correlation, only that it is not always the simple answer. The answer to the question of the genetics question may be epigenetics. The Endocrine Society's research has shown that EDCs effects can be passed to subsequent generations through epigenetic modifications.

High Fructose Corn Syrup I prefer to believe the evidence. If you look at the statistics of obesity and diabetes, you will notice that after 1972 when food became even more processed, and most packaged foods had added high-fructose corn syrup (HFCS is a very cheap sweetener), obesity and diabetes have skyrocketed!

What is the cause of obesity and diabetes and other fatal diseases? It is my contention that added sugar, highly processed foods and carbohydrates are to blame. Along with ECDs the idea of a low fat diet has made us disease ridden and FAT!

Glyphosate is a broad-spectrum herbicide used to kill weeds and grasses. Monsanto says it is safe because humans do not have Shikimate pathway as plants. This pathway affects the metabolic route in plants. However, the human gut bacteria does and can be affected by glyphosate.

Aluminum - Article from National Center for Biotechnology Information:

Link between Aluminum and the Pathogenesis of Alzheimer's Disease: The Integration of the Aluminum and Amyloid Cascade Hypotheses.
By Kawahara M, Kato-Negishi M.

Abstract

Whilst being environmentally abundant, aluminum is not essential for life. On the contrary, aluminum is a widely recognized neurotoxin that inhibits more than 200 biologically important functions and causes various adverse effects in plants, animals, and humans. The relationship between aluminum exposure and neurodegenerative diseases, including dialysis encephalopathy, amyotrophic lateral sclerosis and Parkinsonism dementia in the Kii Peninsula and Guam, and Alzheimer's disease (AD) has been suggested. In particular, the link between aluminum and Alzheimer's disease has been the subject of scientific debate for several decades. However, the complex characteristics of aluminum bioavailability make it difficult to evaluate its toxicity and therefore, the relationship remains to be established. Mounting evidence has suggested that significance of oligomerization of β-amyloid protein and neurotoxicity in the molecular mechanism of AD pathogenesis. Aluminum may play crucial roles as a cross-linker in β-amyloid oligomerization. Here, we review the detailed characteristics of aluminum neurotoxicity based on our own studies and the recent literatures. Our aim is to revisit the link between aluminum and AD and to integrate aluminum and amyloid cascade hypotheses in the context of β-amyloid oligomerization and the interactions with other metals. - NCBI (National Center for Biotechnology Information) PMID: 21423554 PMCID: PMC3056430 DOI: 10.4061/2011/276393

Epigenetics

When I was doing research for my book series *The Body Map*, I came across a very interesting science, epigenetics. Epigenetics is a genetic function that has recently been discovered by biologists. This "software" is responsible for directing DNA in a way that accounts for the development of the various cell types in a growing fetus and adults. This process controls DNA expression, based upon many factors, diet, exercise, inheritance and lifestyle. This wonder of science, is known as epigenetics. The epigenetic process explains how things are happening at the cell level but NOT why. At the time of this writing, we still do not know completely what is driving the process.

> "A single gene can potentially code for tens of thousands of different proteins... It's the way in which genes are switched on and off, though, that has turned out to be mind-boggling, with layer after layer of complexity emerging."
>
> - Michael Le Page, *Genome at 10: Information overload* New Scientist Magazine.

All the instructions for building and maintaining the human body are present in your DNA. So when a protein is needed, the software finds the information it needs to build the protein and then transcribes it into a string. This will be translated later by combining amino acids into a string which is then folded into a protein. Epigenetics is the software that can change the access to that data so that it is effectively "turned off or on". The original DNA is not changed only the access to it. All of the trillions of cells in your body have the same DNA, it is the access to that data that changes what happens in any cell type.

This is my story, nothing in this story should be taken as medical advice. Consult your medical professional for your plan!

The epigenetic process affects the phenotype (the physical expression - eye color, skin color, etc.), while not affecting the genotype (DNA). Epigenetic research has shown that environmental factors affect epigenetic expression. The old saying that "you are what you eat" may be truer than we have thought. Diet and exercise do play a part in how genes are switched on and off. Additionally, our parents can also pass on parts of their epigenetics to their offspring. Over time, these "switches" can be turned on and off. This may be the reason that it takes time to reverse the deleterious effects of misguided advice like; low-fat, high-carbohydrate diets.

I grew up on a farm in Iowa. We had fresh fruit, and vegetables, which we grew in our field. We had fresh eggs from our chickens. My father loved to fish so we had an abundance of fresh water fish. We drank whole milk and very little processed foods. Soda bottles were about 8 oz and cost about 10 cents. It was a rare occasion when we went out to eat. There were very few fast-food restaurants in the 50s. In the 60s, many fast-food restaurants began to appear. Back then I was lean and had good health. If you look at the statistics of obesity, heart disease and diabetes, you see a steady increase in instances starting in the 1960s. It was at that point in time that saturated fat and cholesterol were classified as "BAD" and the government and medical community started recommending a low-fat diet.

In the 1950s and 1960s in the United States and Japan, technology was developed to cheaply remove oils from oilseeds (corn, soybean, cottonseed, red palm seeds, etc.)
- Popkin B, Drewnowski A. Dietary fats and the nutrition transition: New trends in the global diet. Nutr Rev. 1997;55:31–43

Between 1985 and 2010 individual intake of vegetable oils increased threefold to sixfold, depending on the subpopulation studied. In China, which has moderate but not high vegetable oil intake, persons age two and older now consume on average almost 300 calories and more than 30 grams of vegetable oil daily
- Popkin BM. Will China's nutrition transition overwhelm its health care system and slow economic growth? Health Aff (Millwood) 2008;27:1064–1076.

It is said that some of the epigenetic markers do get passed on to the next generation, but that would require additional research outside the scope of this book.

America is the most obese country in the world (36%+ of the population) eating a diet of low-fat and high carbohydrates as directed by the health industry. If the guidelines do not work, why do people continue to try to follow it? The answer is; the blame is not put on the guideline but on the person following the guideline. It is your fault that it did not work; you did not follow it closely enough. Most people then just give up!

I clearly remember the low-fat craze (still going on today). As a result, people thought that the fact that a food was low fat, they could eat as much as they wanted. The thing about carbohydrate consumption is that it does not satisfy, so you tend to need more and more. Look at soda, it contains massive amounts of sodium and sugar. This is not designed to quench your thirst like the advertisements imply, no; that combination actually makes you want more soda. Why do you think that convenience stores came up with the 64 oz serving, all of that for less than a $1? The drug companies are elated because they will sell more statins and diabetes drugs. The food companies are pleased because they will sell more of their toxic swill. The diet companies are joyful because they will sell more programs as the population swells with obesity. The health clubs and fitness gurus are grateful because they will sell more memberships as the citizenry struggle to take off surplus weight put on by excess sugar. The result is that we get sicker, and they get wealthier! When will this cycle end?

If you are obese or have nutritional illnesses like diabetes, I hope by now you are getting the idea that the recommendations prevalent in today's world simply do not work. Change in our health will only come when we change our approach. Appendix B has a list of medical professionals who have proven results in improving the health of their patients. They can help you make the choices that will ultimately improve your health and life.

Inflammation, Free Radicals and Oxidative Stress

One thing that is not obvious from the surface is the damage done by oxidation, inflammation and free radicals. It is oxidation of the lipid proteins that form the "bad" LDL. Those damaged lipoproteins get outside the artery. The immune system is engaged, and it tries to clean up the aberrant molecules which inadvertently caused more issues. The old illustration of grease building up in the walls of your blood stream is not accurate. It may seem logical to think of it that way, but that is still way off the mark.

Let's start by explaining what inflammation is and what it does. Inflammation can be good, and it can be bad. When the body experiences an infectious or toxic invader or some type of traumatic event, the general purpose of inflammation is to protect the site from further damage. This inflammation is often accompanied by pain of some type. Examples of this type of inflammation are: arthritis, pancreatitis, appendicitis, asthma and pneumonia. However, the inflammation we are concerned about in this book is deadly silent until an event causes pain or death.

Inflammation involving the lining of the blood vessels and organs is our concern because it causes heart disease, atherosclerosis, a stroke, kidney disease and other serious illnesses.

Some foods that create inflammation include:
- Refined vegetable oils (canola oil, soybean oils - high in pro-inflammatory omega-6 fatty acids)
- Refined carbohydrates including grains
- Added sugars
- Trans fats
- Hydrogenated fats
- Pasteurized dairy

Some foods are anti-inflammatory.
- Healthy fats: grass-fed beef, grass-fed butter
- Wild fish
- Eggs from free range chickens
- Dark green leafy vegetables
- Whole fruit - berries etc.
- Red wine / dark chocolate (NO SUGAR)

PROCESSES

Free Radicals

> FREE RADICALS
>
> "A free radical can be defined as any molecular species capable of independent existence that contains an unpaired electron in an atomic orbital. The presence of an unpaired electron results in certain common properties that are shared by most radicals. Many radicals are unstable and highly reactive. They can either donate an electron to or accept an electron from other molecules, therefore behaving as oxidants or reductants. The most important oxygen-containing free radicals in many disease states are hydroxyl radical, superoxide anion radical, hydrogen peroxide, oxygen singlet, hypochlorite, nitric oxide radical, and peroxynitrite radical. These are highly reactive species, capable in the nucleus, and in the membranes of cells of damaging biologically relevant molecules such as DNA, proteins, carbohydrates, and lipids. Free radicals attack important macromolecules leading to cell damage and homeostatic disruption. Targets of free radicals include all kinds of molecules in the body. Among them, lipids, nucleic acids, and proteins are the major targets."
>
> -Lobo, V et al. "Free radicals, antioxidants and functional foods: Impact on human health." Pharmacognosy reviews vol. 4,8 (2010): 118-26. doi:10.4103/0973-7847.70902

Free radicals want to balance their electrons, so they will steal an electron from another molecule. When this cascades to several molecules, it will cause oxidative stress. Free radicals come from internal and external sources. External sources include smoking, radiation, and even exercise.

When you have an excess of oxidative stress, many diseases generally follow, these diseases can include diabetes and cancer.

Glutathione (GSH) is a powerful antioxidant which has been shown to reduce oxidative stress. This molecule is created in the cells and requires three amino acids: glutamine, glycine, and cysteine to manufacture it.

However, it is said that ingesting glutathione in pill form has very little benefit.

"Aging is associated with a diminished capacity to make glutathione," said Dr. Rajagopal V. Sekhar, associate professor of medicine - endocrinology at Baylor College of Medicine

Dr. Sekhar goes on to say that when glutathione levels are low, oxidative stress can increase. Their research showed that a deficiency of glutathione also impaired fat-burning.

"When we give these older people cysteine and glycine in their diets and corrected glutathione deficiency, amazingly their fat oxidation also normalized," he said. "The older people go back to burning fat as well as younger people within 14 days." - *Correcting glutathione deficiency improves impaired mitochondrial fat burning, insulin resistance in aging.* - Dr. Rajagopal V. Sekhar, associate professor of medicine - endocrinology at Baylor College of Medicine

Glutathione is also partly responsible for apoptosis. Apoptosis is the process of programmed cell death. If the cell cannot die and be disposed of by macrophages, it becomes a cancer. Cancer is the uncontrolled cell growth. Glutathione is also critical for detoxification.

"Essentially Glutathione is a magnet, passing through each of our cells, gathering up toxins and heavy metals in order to purge them from the body. Once a Glutathione molecule gathers up these toxins, it is converted into its oxidized form Glutathione Disulfide (GSSG)". - Jimmy Gutman - http://glutathionepro.com/

Where do we get glutathione? The cells manufacture glutathione from amino acids (Cysteine, Glutamic acid and Glycine). When the amino acids are not in adequate supply, then glutathione is not produced in the amount required for good health, and the problems begin. Is it any surprise that we get the required amino acids from meat, egg yolks, unpasteurized milk and other unpasteurized dairy, the very thing that the nutritionists say to avoid? No wonder we have an increase in disease! Glutathione can also be found in vegetables like avocados, asparagus, broccoli, kale, garlic, onions, cauliflower and walnuts.

Autophagy (sounds like: 'a tof a gee')

Autophagy is the "cleaning lady" for the body, it is a process whereby the p62 protein recognizes toxic cellular waste and starts the process of scavenging the abhorrent cells. This process prevents a disease from spreading further. The body improves its health as the damaged cells are removed.

In order to start the autophagy process one way is to go on a low carbohydrate/ good fats diet (LCHF). The LCHF diet keeps you from getting hungry so you can effectively do intermittent fasting. Carbohydrates are broken down to glycogen and stored in the muscles, and liver so energy can be released quickly. There is limited space for glycogen, when it becomes full, the excess is stored in the adipose (fat) cells. When the glycogen levels fall the body turns to fat stores for energy.

Autophagy can be responsible for eliminating damaged DNA in the cell. The absence of this process can lead to an occurrence of cancer. Cancer happens when damaged cells refuse to die. Apoptosis (programmed cell death) works with autophagy. When cells die graciously, the autophagy process cleans up the mess.

C-reactive protein (CRP)

When inflammation is present in the body, a simple blood test will show an increase of this protein. When the body discovers a certain level of inflammation, the liver makes this protein. The more CRP you have in the blood the higher the level of inflammation. Increased levels of CRP have been linked to Obesity, diabetes, smoking and gum disease. CRP is produced by the liver.

> **What are the causes of elevated C-reactive protein?**
>
> "Elevated CRP can signal many different conditions, including cancer, cardiovascular disease, infection, and autoimmune conditions such as rheumatoid arthritis, lupus, and inflammatory bowel disease. The chronic inflammation behind an elevated CRP level may also be influenced by genetics, a sedentary lifestyle, too much stress, and exposure to environmental toxins such as secondhand tobacco smoke. Diet has a huge impact, particularly one that contains a lot of refined, processed and manufactured foods." - Dr. Andrew Weil

Mitochondria

Life stops without energy in the form of ATP. Every cell in the body, except neurons have multiple upon multiples of ATP producing machines. Without a continuous supply of ATP major health problems begin. The next chapter has more detail.

> "The supply of ATP must be steady because its lack would kill an organism in a matter of minutes. Poisons like cyanide kill so quickly by blocking processing of ATP". *ATP: The Perfect Energy Currency for the Cell* by Jerry Bergman, CRSQ Vol 36(1) June, 1999
>
> "One central coenzyme is adenosine triphosphate (ATP), the universal energy currency of cells. There is only a small amount of ATP in cells, but as it is continuously regenerated, **the human body can use about its own weight in ATP per day."** Dimroth P, von Ballmoos C, Meier T (March 2006). *"Catalytic and mechanical cycles in F-ATP synthases. Fourth in the Cycles Review Series".*

Sodium Potassium Pumps - The body's electrical system. The next chapter has more detail.

NAFLD Non-Alcohol Fatty Liver Disease (without evidence of liver damage) and there is also a condition known as Non-Alcoholic Steatohepatitis (NASH). It is estimated that 67% of the obese have a fatty liver. Over time where there is too much glucose, too much insulin the result is a fatty liver. However, know that there are those known as TOFI (Thin on the outside fat on the inside) who are diabetic and have a fatty liver not associated with alcohol.

Removing excess visceral fat by liposuction does not solve the problem. Liposuction does not remove the fat in the liver and does not solve the metabolic issue. The liver can only store a certain amount of glycogen when it has as much as it can handle the rest is turned into fat. A function known as de novo lipogenesis (DNL) is a process that converts excess glycogen to fat. It is then exported to the adipose cells.

The body also has a reverse process called gluconeogenesis. This process takes stored fat and glycogen and releases it for energy.

The liver packages cholesterol and fat (triglycerides) in the form of Very-low-density lipoprotein (VLDL). The VLDLs are put in the blood stream to be sent to the cells. See the next chapter about cholesterol.

A blood test can check for an enzyme called gamma-glutamyl transpeptidase (GGT) — this test can tell you if your liver, kidneys or pancreas is in danger.

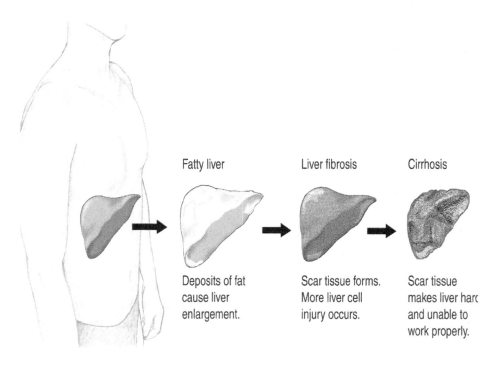

Fatty liver	Liver fibrosis	Cirrhosis
Deposits of fat cause liver enlargement.	Scar tissue forms. More liver cell injury occurs.	Scar tissue makes liver harc and unable to work properly.

How do the cells get energy from food?

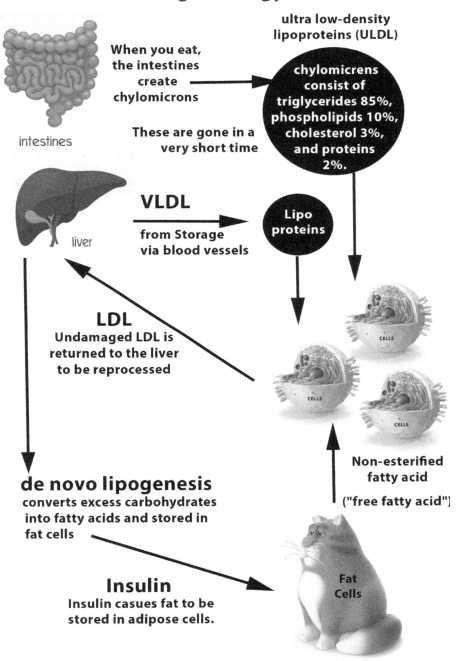

ultra low-density
lipoproteins (ULDL)

When you eat,
the intestines
create
chylomicrons

**chylomicrens
consist of
triglycerides 85%,
phospholipids 10%,
cholesterol 3%,
and proteins
2%.**

intestines

These are gone in a
very short time

liver

VLDL

**from Storage
via blood vessels**

Lipo
proteins

LDL
**Undamaged LDL is
returned to the liver
to be reprocessed**

CELLS

CELLS

CELLS

Non-esterified
fatty acid

("free fatty acid")

de novo lipogenesis
**converts excess carbohydrates
into fatty acids and stored in
fat cells**

Insulin
**Insulin casues fat to be
stored in adipose cells.**

Fat
Cells

The much publicized diets with emphasis solely on calories are fallacious. It is excess carbohydrates and not calories only that make a fat man fat. The tiresome business of totting up daily calories, on which most modern reducing diets are based, is a waste of time for an obese person. Because, as Professor Kekwick and Dr. Pawan showed, a fat man may maintain his weight on a low-calorie diet, if it is taken mainly as carbohydrate, but he will lose weight on a much higher calorie diet provided he eats it mainly in the form of fat and protein. - *Eat Fat And Grow Slim* - Richard MacKarness, M.B., B.S (1958)

V

Misunderstood Chemistry in the Body: Cholesterol & Fat

"Dying with 'corrected' Cholesterol is not a successful outcome"
- John Abramson, M.D. Harvard University

"In 1964…the famous Houston heart surgeon Michael DeBakey reported similarly negative findings from the records on seventeen hundred of his own patients. And even if high cholesterol was associated with an increased incidence of heart disease, this begged the question of why so many people, as Gofman had noted in Science, suffer coronary heart disease despite having low cholesterol, and why a tremendous number of people with high cholesterol never get heart disease or die of it"
- Gary Taubes - *Good Calorie Bad Calorie,*

Eating fat does NOT make you fat! It is what gets turned into fat and stored. Stored fat comes mostly from carbohydrates.

While saturated fats may increase the LDL cholesterol (the so-called bad cholesterol) levels in your body, it does not increase the cardiovascular mortality rate. And not all LDLs are the same. Saturated fats increase the HDL cholesterol (The so-called good cholesterol) which would be a good thing. However, the inverse is also true, that eating fewer saturated fats does cause higher mortality rates. We could site multiple research studies that show that saturated fats do not increase your chances of getting heart disease or diabetes.

Does cholesterol cause heart disease? You first must understand what cholesterol is and what it does in the body.

According to the Weston Price Foundation (westonprice.org) The highest concentration of cholesterol is found in the brain. Research has found that seniors with the high cholesterol have better memories. Cholesterol plays many roles The Weston Price Foundation continues and says it is accountable for regulating serotonin in the brain. A lack of serotonin is said to be responsible for controlling sleep, it supports blood clotting, bone health, sexual function, mood disorders, anxiety and depression. I hope you are getting the idea that the body is a very complex machine, there are so many processes dependent on each other that one-size fits all approach would be foolish.

From a talk by Mary Fallon
*The Oiling of Americ*a

Deaths from Myocardial Infarction (MI)
(Heart Attack)

1921 - First recorded incident of MI
1930 - 3,000 deaths recorded from MI
1960 - 500,000 deaths recorded from MI

I came across an article by Lisa Nelson RD, *Cholesterol Too Low*. I asked her if I could include it in the book. She graciously allowed me to publish this article, you can find her at: http://www.lisanelsonrd.com, please visit her site.

"Cholesterol is often viewed as "bad" these days and many people are doing everything they can to lower cholesterol levels as much as possible. This isn't necessarily a good thing.

Cholesterol is essential for many normal bodily functions. Enzymes use cholesterol to produce vitamin D, steroid hormones (estrogen, progesterone, testosterone), stress hormones, and bile acids for digestion. Cholesterol forms a membrane that surrounds all cells and is also a critical part of regenerating damaged endothelial cells (inner layer of blood vessel walls).

For most individuals, if you do not eat enough dietary cholesterol the liver produces the cholesterol needed for bodily functions. The amount of cholesterol in your diet determines how much the liver produces.

Cholesterol is essential for optimal health and pushing levels too low can cause problems. Back in 1994, the American Heart Association issued a statement noting an increase in deaths from trauma, cancer, hemorrhagic stroke, respiratory diseases, and infectious diseases in individuals with cholesterol levels less than 160 mg/dl. It's worth noting that a large number of these deaths seemed to be due to poor health unrelated to the low cholesterol levels.

However, since then many studies are linking low cholesterol levels with depression, suicide, impulsive, aggression, and anxiety when levels drop below 160 mg/dl. One psychologist suggested having too low cholesterol alters brain cell function and the brain cells with low cholesterol levels may have fewer receptors for the mood-elevating neurotransmitter serotonin. This could be the reason low cholesterol levels increase rates of depression.

With the rapidly rising use of medications, such as statin drugs, I'm noticing individuals reporting cholesterol levels that are dropping into potentially dangerous territory. Work with your physician to ensure you maintain healthy cholesterol levels appropriate for you."

We have already seen that cholesterol is necessary for sex hormones, cell membranes and nerve tissue. Not all LDL cholesterol is the same. Initially LDL cholesterol, inside of the Lipid Protein molecules, is large and floats happily along in the blood stream and delivers its cargo where it is needed. If the LDL molecules are attacked by free radicals or oxidation, they can become small and dense. These can cause inflammation and begin to enter the walls of the arteries. What is not usually revealed in blood tests is the amount of large buoyant LDL and small dense LDL. What should be tested is the triglyceride/HDL ratio which is a better determinant of health issues.

Cholesterol is made by all the cells in our bodies except neurons. It is said that we create more than four times as much cholesterol than we eat. The body attempts to maintain homeostasis by making cholesterol when there is a lack of it. When we eat meat, the cells produce less cholesterol. Because of our God-given design, it is difficult to reduce cholesterol on our own. The question is, if we are designed to manufacture cholesterol when it is perceived to be too low and cholesterol is necessary for life in many ways, why would we want to lower it artificially? I could speculate, but I will simply say that people think they know better than the designer. They build their theory of how the body should operate based on the faulty idea

that we evolved and our design is open to modification. I don't want to get too far off the subject of this publication, but the idea that this marvelous machine was built by chance mutations is foolish nonsense! Equally as

110

important is the fact that a massive number of functions that are critical for our existence must be operational all at the same time or life cannot continue. I am writing a series of books that look at the human body, and its operation called The Body Map Series. In that series, I have a detailed description of each part of the human anatomy and how it operates starting at a microbiological level. The extremely slow process of evolution is NOT a viable explanation for our existence. The body was clearly designed by a creator however you characterize creation.

What does cholestrol provide to our bodies?

"Every cell in the human body, besides neurons, can produce cholesterol. On average your body will produce roughly 2000mg of cholesterol a day. That's approximately a dozen eggs worth of cholesterol. Even that number doesn't fully embrace the true scope of the amount of cholesterol in our bodies. Taking an average cholesterol value of 200 mg per dL, with an average blood volume of 5 to 7 liters, this equates to 10,000 to 14,000 mg of circulating cholesterol"
- Mary Enig - *Know Your Fats* Published by Bethesda Press.

Cholesterol is shuttled around the body inside of a lipoprotein. Since the blood is "watery" and cholesterol is "fatty" it must have a way to be transported through the blood (oil and water do not mix). This transport is initially characterized as big and fluffy when it starts out. As the cholesterol is delivered to the cells, it becomes smaller and more dense. This is not a problem, unless it is attacked by oxidation or free radicals. In this case, the LDL (lipoprotein) will not be recognized by the liver receptors and will be refused entry. These aberrant LDL particles float around in the blood and can cause problems. If there is a mutation on one of the chromosomes, 19 base pares at position p13.2 the person will be classified as familial hypercholesterolemia. The mutation of that gene will result in liver receptors not being able to recycle the cholesterol in the lipoprotein.

"Low-density lipoprotein receptors play a critical role in regulating the amount of cholesterol in the blood. They are particularly abundant in the liver, which is the organ responsible for removing most excess cholesterol from the body. The number of low-density lipoprotein receptors on the surface of liver cells determines how quickly cholesterol (in the form of low-density lipoproteins) is removed from the bloodstream". - https://ghr.nlm.nih.gov/gene/LDLR#location

Cytogenetic Location: 19p13.2, which is the short (p) arm of <u>chromosome 19</u> at position 13.2

Molecular Location: base pairs 11,089,362 to 11,133,830 on chromosome 19 (Homo sapiens Updated Annotation Release 109.20190607, GRCh38.p13) (<u>NCBI</u>)

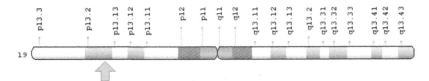

https://ghr.nlm.nih.gov/gene/LDLR#location

Cells are surrounded by lipid bilayer. Cholesterol in this bilayer can increase or decrease. When cholesterol is increased membrane access is restricted. When cholesterol is decreased membrane access is increased. This is critical for the operation of the sodium/potassium pump because it keeps Na+ (sodium) and K+ (potassium) from leaking across the membrane. If cholesterol were not present, more energy would be required to pull the ions back against the concentration gradient. (see the description of the Sodium/potassium pump below)

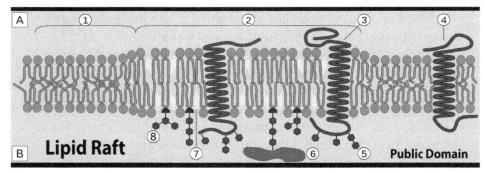

Wikipedia contributors. "Lipid raft." Wikipedia, The Free Encyclopedia, 27 Jul. 2019. Web. 3 Aug. 2019.

[A] Intracellular space or cytosol
[B] Extracellular space or vesicle/Golgi apparatus lumen

1-Non-raft membrane
2-Lipid raft
3-Lipid raft associated transmembrane protein
4-Non-raft membrane protein
5-Glycosylation modifications (on glycoproteins and glycolipids)
6-GPI-anchored protein

7-Cholesterol
8-Glycolipid

The Sodium/Potassium pump
The Electric Generator

Another system critical to life is the sodium-potassium pump. Your ability to hear, see, think, feel, and move your muscle depends on this pump. The pump is an active transport for moving potassium and sodium ions in and out of the cell membrane to create a voltage across the cell membrane. It is considered an active transport, because it uses energy in the form of ATP to accomplish its objective, in contrast to diffusion of oxygen, carbon dioxide, and osmosis of water, which is a passive transport. The pump can be found in virtually every cell in the body. It is estimated that 1/3 of the body's energy is used for this process. In an article about the pump it states:

> "As one measure of their importance, it has been estimated that roughly 25% of all cytoplasmic ATP is hydrolyzed by sodium pumps in resting humans. In nerve cells, approximately 70% of the ATP is consumed to fuel sodium pumps.
> - Laura Austgen,
> http://www.vivo.colostate.edu/hbooks/molecules/sodium_pump.html

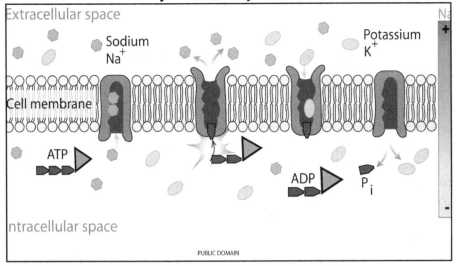

In a resting state the difference in positively charged sodium ions (Na$^+$) on the outside of the cell membrane and positively charged potassium ions (K$^+$) on the inside create an voltage inside the cell of approximately -70 to -80 mv. It also takes energy to maintain the resting state.

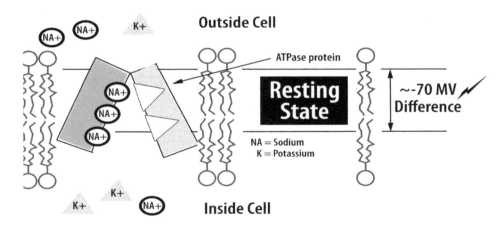

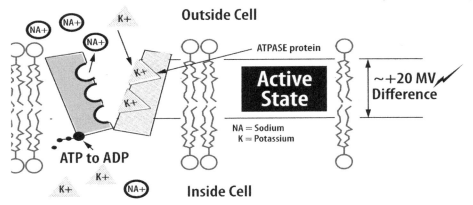

A stimulus (electrical or chemical), causes the sodium gates to open in the cell membrane, and the sodium ions begin to move in. This short-circuits the cell and the voltage drops, creating the action potential. (Action potentials also called an impulse or 'spike') This change in voltage is sent through the nerve and muscle cells in a wave action across neighboring cells to the destination. These waves only move in one direction because the gates are closed and will only open for a short period of time. Otherwise, the action would move back in the opposite direction. (A wonderful feat of God's engineering.)

Nerve cells are poor conductors, requiring the voltage to be maintained all the way to the destination. Since communication is digital (meaning frequency not amplitude) the more intense the event (the louder sound for instance), the more action potentials occur per second. This action potential is an "all or nothing response." If stimulation exceeds the threshold, an impulse will be generated if it does not meet the threshold, the action potential will not be put into motion.

There are three phases in this process:

1. Depolarization - where the sodium ion gate opens and sodium ions rush in causing a change in voltage from -70 mv to +20 to +40 mv the inside is now positively charged.

2. Re-polarization - potassium ion gate opens and now Potassium rush to outside of the cell.

3. <u>Recovery/Refractory Period</u> - Sodium ions are now

> pumped out of the cell and potassium ions are brought
> back in. Three sodium ions are pumped out for every
> two potassium ions coming in.

This is not an exhaustive description of the pump. This pump must exist, or life at the cell ends and nerve impulses never reach their destination. The body is a system of collaborating parts that are so interrelated, that it would be impossible for these parts to operate on their own. ATP generates energy for the cell, without ATP you would quickly die. Sodium-potassium pumps consume a very significant amount of ATP doing its job, showing how critical this function is to life. Without ATP energy, the body dies, without the electrical energy created from the sodium-potassium pump the body does not function.

When an event or events happen at a nerve cell, this causes an action to take place. However, it must reach a threshold before action is taken. You should be asking how does the nerve cell determine what is enough to cause an action and how would a cell know that?

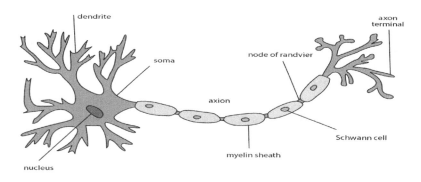

An insulator over the axion will speed up the signal. This insulator is known as the myelin sheath. The sheath does not have voltage-gated ion channels; this maintains a separation of the charge between the interior and exterior of the cell. However, sodium diffuses along the axion. If the myelin sheath were too long, the signal would be very weak when it reached the next segment. God's design is astonishing, every so often there is a break in the sheath, called the nodes of Ranvier. These are spaced at about every one mm or so, and contain large amounts of voltage-gated sodium channels, and allow enough sodium into the axon to regenerate the action potential.

> "Each time the action potential reaches a node of Ranvier, it is restored to its original action potential (+35mV)". Kenneth S. Saladin, *Anatomy & physiology: the unity of form and function.* 6th ed. McGraw-Hill

This process of recharging is known as saltatory conduction (from the Latin saltare, to hop or leap.

ATP synthase - The Power source

Adenosine triphosphate (ATP)

Adenosine diphosphate (ADP)

Adenosine triphosphate, also is known as ATP is a complex fundamental energy currency for all life. ATP is so critical for life to exist that the lack of it will kill you in a matter of minutes.

Above is a chemical diagram of ATP and ADP. The darker area is ADP the result of one ATP being used.

> "The supply of ATP must be steady because its lack would kill an organism in a matter of minutes. Poisons like cyanide kill so quickly by blocking processing of ATP according to Bergman". *ATP: The Perfect Energy Currency for the Cell by* Jerry Bergman, CRSQ Vol 36(1) June, 1999.

Excuse me if I stop and praise God! Sometimes, I am emotionally overwhelmed by his magnificence. After writing the previous paragraph, I am awestruck. Do you realize how far He is above all others? He is truly worthy of praise. I am perplexed, that anyone would dare suggest that any of this happened by mere chance it is an insult to all thinking humans. I like what Psalm 139:14 says

> *"I will praise thee; for I am fearfully [and] wonderfully made: marvellous [are] thy works; and [that] my soul knoweth right well".*

> "One central coenzyme is adenosine triphosphate (ATP), the universal energy currency of cells. There is only a small amount of ATP in cells, but as it is continuously regenerated, **the human body can use about its weight in ATP per day."** Dimroth P, von Ballmoos C, Meier T (March 2006). "*Catalytic and mechanical cycles in F-ATP synthases. Fourth in the Cycles Review Series*".

The total human body content of ATP is only about 50 grams, which must constantly be recycled every day. The ultimate source of energy for constructing ATP is food; ATP is simply the carrier and regulation-storage unit of energy. The average daily intake of 2,500 food calories translates into a turnover of a whopping 180 kg (400 lbs) of ATP Kornberg, 1989. *For the love of enzymes.* Harvard University Press. Cambridge, MA (Kornberg, 1989, p. 65).

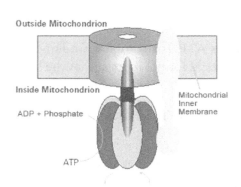

Outside Mitochondrion

Inside Mitochondrion

ADP + Phosphate

Mitochondrial Inner Membrane

ATP

The mitochondria is an organelle found in eukaryotic (cells with a nucleus) cells that perform cellular respiration among other things. Cellular respiration is a series of chemical reactions through which glucose is converted into the energy carrier - ATP. The mitochondria have its own genome (mtDNA). This is separate and distinct from the DNA found in the nucleus. This mtDNA originates only from your mother.

There is more going on in the mitochondria, but we will focus on the ATP synthase. ATP is generated by converting the ADP molecule, (adenosine diphosphate) by adding a third phosphate unit. The ATP synthase has a wheel-like structure that turns up to 200 times per second and produces three ATP molecules on each turn, resulting in six hundred new ATPs per second. Each cell is estimated to have about one billion ATP molecules at any one time. However, this is only enough to last a few minutes and ADP is recycled to ATP continuously.

You need ATP to move your muscles among many other things. ATP is not stable enough to be sent to the muscle through the blood so it must be available at the cell level. It is incredible that there are many of these molecular machines manufacturing ATP 24/7. It takes ATP to make ATP so the question we need to ask the evolutionist is: "How did life exist before ATP?"

> "How could life survive without ATP since no form of life we know of today can do that?" and "How could ATP evolve and where are the many transitional forms required to evolve the complex ATP molecule?" No feasible candidates exist and none can exist because only a perfect ATP molecule can properly carry out its role in the cell." *ATP: The Perfect Energy Currency for the Cell,* CRSQ Volume 36(1) June 1999, Jerry Bergman

> The ATP synthase molecule is composed of thirty-one component proteins. Without any part of this it would not work and the cell would have no energy source to function. Both the ATP and the ATP synthase are coded for by the genetic information built into the DNA. - David Rosevear, *Interpreting Origins Science*

ATP is necessary for the creation of ATP and many other processes. Active cell transport (moving molecules in and out of the cell), muscle contraction, the formation of proteins, chemical reactions, maintenance of the Na/K pump (Sodium-potassium pump), action potential signaling and transporting molecules across the cell.

Creating ATP is not a simple process, and that is an understatement. The raw material (a six carbon glucose) goes through multiple processes to get to the end product. There are three processes: Glycolysis, The Krebs

Cycle and finally the Electron Transport chain. This process requires many specialized enzymes to make ATP. The output of the process is CO2 (Carbon Dioxide) + H20 (water) + ATP (energy) ~ 34-38 molecules. For more detail see my book *The Body Map - Designed from the Beginning.*

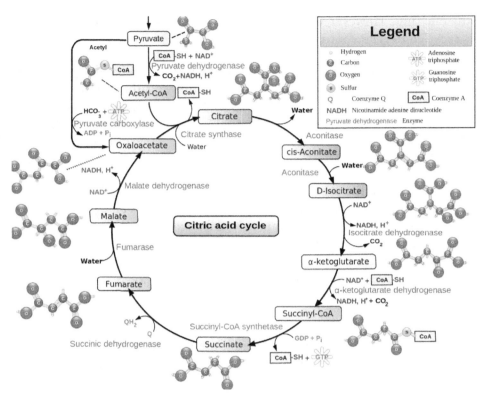

At any one moment in time you generally only have six seconds of available ATP. This energy MUST be replaced continually or the body dies this is why cyanide kills so fast!

The following is a digest from a presentation
by David Diamond, PhD. Biology - a Neuroscientist
[indicates my comments]

The Diet Heart Hypothesis fallacy:

Dietary Saturated Fat => Increase Serum Cholestrol => Cardiovascular Disease

"We propose that carbohydrate-induced lipodemia [*fat in the blood*] is a common phenomenon, especially in areas of the world distinguished by caloric abundance and obesity"- Association of American Physicians 1961

===

Ancel Keys B.A. Economics, PhD Fish Physiology - [*his 1961 fallacy based on bad science, faulty research and the deceitful practice of selecting only data that supported his hypothesis.*]

"Americans eat too much fat... and most of that is saturated fat - the insidious kind that increases blood cholestrol, damages arteries and leads to coronary disease." [*not necessarily true*]

"The only sure way to control blood cholestrol is to reduce fat in the U.S. diet from 40% to 15% of total calories and cut saturated fat from 17% to 4% of total calories." [*this has proven to be a disaster for millions of people*]

American Heart Association: From their website: https://www.heart.org Limit saturated fat and trans fat and replace them with the better fats, mono-unsaturated and polyunsaturated. If you need to lower your blood cholesterol, reduce saturated fat to no more than 5 to 6 percent of total calories. For someone eating 2,000 calories a day, that's about 13 grams of saturated fat. [*accessed 5/20/19*]

[*better research accessed 5/20/19*]
www.**nutritioncoalition.us**/saturated-fats-do-they-cause-heart-disease/
The Disputed Science on Saturated Fats - Summary of the data: "The rigorous trial data do not support the allegation that saturated fats cause cardiovascular mortality or total mortality. While saturated fats can be shown to raise the "bad" LDL-cholesterol, this elevated risk factor does not result in higher mortality rates, very likely reflecting a more complicated pathway for cardiovascular disease than simply LDL-C (i.e., saturated fats also consistently raise the "good" HDL-cholesterol, which may be a compensating effect).

Regarding the observational evidence, meta-analyses of this data consistently find no association between saturated fat and cardiovascular disease. Moreover, there is a substantial observational finding that low consumption of saturated fats is associated with higher mortality and higher rates of stroke."

Misunderstood Chemistry In The Body

In 1908, M.A. Ignatovsky fed high-fat protein-rich animal products to a group of rabbits. The result was: the rabbits developed something like cardiovascular disease. His hypothesis was that high-fat diets cause heart disease. There is only one problem with his prognosis, rabbits are strictly herbivores! Their God-given design is not meant to process meat in their diet. Dr. Uffe Ravnskov in his book The Cholestrol Myth explains that the deposits found in the rabbits are not the same as in humans with atherosclerosis.

Dr. Kilmer McCully in his book The Heart Revolution: The Extraordinary Discovery That Finally Laid The Cholestrol Myth to Rest points out that it is Homosysteine an amino acid in our body that is linked to heart disease, blood clots and stroke. Keeping homosysteine in check can be accomplished by adequate levels of B6, B12 and Folic acid from whole foods. He goes on to point out that when the food manufactures process and refine their products it destroys the B vitamins necessary for good health.

"Fat is the caloric reserve material of nature. The whale stores fat in his subcutaneous layers against the rigors of life at the Pole, the camel stores it in his hump against hard times in the desert, the African sheep stores it in his tail and his buttocks against the day when even the parched grass shall have withered away. But fats are more than stores of reserve caloric material. They are heat insulators, they are fillers of dead spaces, and they are facilitators of movement in rigid compartments such as the orbit, the pelvis, and the capsules of joints. They are also essential building materials. Animal fats contain three groups of substances: the neutral fats which are chiefly energy providers, the lipids containing phosphorus that enter into most tissues and bulk largely in the brain and the central nervous system, and the sterols that are the basis of most hormones.

The body must have proteins and animal fats. It has no need for carbohydrates, and, given the two essential foodstuffs, it can get all the calories it needs from them."

- Foreword by Sir Heneage Ogilvie *Eat Fat & Grow Slim* (1958)

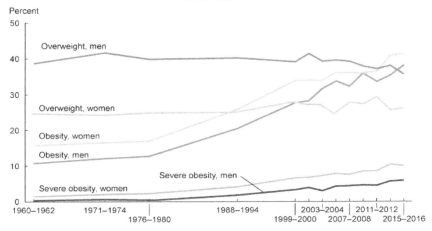

Figure. Trends in overweight, obesity, and severe obesity among men and women aged 20–74: United States, 1960–1962 through 2015–2016

NOTES: Data are age adjusted by the direct method to U.S. Census 2000 estimates using age groups 20–39, 40–59, and 60–74. Overweight is body mass index (BMI) of 25.0–29.9 kg/m²; obesity is BMI at or above 30.0 kg/m²; and severe obesity is BMI at or above 40.0 kg/m². Pregnant women are excluded from the analysis.
SOURCES: NCHS, National Health Examination Survey and National Health and Nutrition Examination Surveys.

You should note that when the guidelines for a good diet were introduced, reduce saturated fat and increase carbohydrates the level of obesity has risen dramatically. The chart below has the percentages of over weight to severely obese from 1960 to 2016.

Year	% overweight	% Obese	% Severely Obese
1960–1962	31.5	**13.4**	**0.9**
1971–1974	32.7	14.5	1.3
1976–1980	32.1	15.0	1.4
1988–1994	32.6	23.2	3.0
1999–2000	33.6	30.9	5.0
2001–2002	34.4	31.2	5.4
2003–2004	33.4	32.9	5.1
2005–2006	32.2	35.1	6.2
2007–2008	33.6	34.3	6.0
2009–2010	32.7	36.1	6.6
2011–2012	33.3	35.3	6.6
2013–2014	31.9	38.2	8.1
2015–2016	31.0	**40.0**	**8.0**
		+26.6%	**+7.1%**
		~3 times	~ 8 times More

123

SOURCES: NCHS, National Health Examination Survey and National Health and Nutrition Examination Survey. For details see: https://www.cdc.gov/nchs/data/hestat/obesity_adult_15_16/obesity_adult_15_16.htm

> *Reminder: I am researching the issues; I am not a licensed doctor and do not practice medicine. You need to contact a practitioner who has the right to diagnose and treat your issue, see appendix B for a list of practitioners.*

Statins

Statins are proclaimed to be the savior of us all by lowering cholesterol. However, the drug industry has inflated the benefits of the drug.

> Business Week Cover Story, January 17, 2008
> **Do Cholesterol Drugs Do Any Good?**
>
> Research suggests that, except among high-risk heart patients, the benefits of statins such as Lipitor are overstated. The second crucial point is hiding in plain sight in Pfizer's own Lipitor newspaper ad. The dramatic 36% figure has an asterisk. **Read the smaller type. It says**: "That means in a large clinical study, 3% of patients taking a sugar pill or placebo had a heart attack compared to 2% of patients taking Lipitor."
>
> *That means only a 1% reduction NOT 36% as implied!*

The question we must ask first is: Do we need to reduce our cholesterol levels to avoid a heart attack? Were you aware that statins lower essential coQ10 needed for the generation of energy in the cell? Statins actually increase the number of lipoprotein receptors on the liver allowing it to take in more LDL? This shows up in a blood test. However, statins still do not take in the small dense LDL which has been damaged by free radicals! The damaged small dense LDL is associated with blockage!

Most Heart Attack Patients' Cholesterol Levels Did Not Indicate Cardiac Risk
Date: January 13, 2009 Source: University of California - Los Angeles
Summary:
A new national study has shown that nearly 75 percent of patients hospitalized for a heart attack had cholesterol levels that would indicate they were not at high risk for a cardiovascular event, according to current national cholesterol guidelines.

We have already discovered that cholesterol is critical in many functions of the human body, and cholesterol is not the main cause of atheroscleroses.

The issue for me, other than the inflated claims of the statin drug, is: are there side effects? YES!

Reminder: I am researching the issues; I am not a licensed doctor and do not practice medicine. You need to contact a practitioner who has the right to diagnose and treat your issue, see appendix B for a list of practitioners.

FDA Safety Announcement:

The statin drug labels have been revised to provide patients with more information on the safe and effective use of statins. Patients should be aware of the following information:

There have been rare reports of **serious liver problems** in patients taking statins. Patients should notify their healthcare professional right away if they have the following symptoms: unusual fatigue or weakness; loss of appetite; upper belly pain; dark-colored urine; or yellowing of the skin or the whites of the eyes.

Memory loss and confusion have been reported with statin use. These reported events were generally not serious and went away once the drug was no longer being taken.

Increases in blood sugar levels have been reported with statin use.

https://www.fda.gov/drugs/drug-safety-and-availability/fda-drug-safety-communication-important-safety-label-changes-cholesterol-lowering-statin-drugs.

We are also aware that the most common side effect of statin use is muscle pain. There are many other reported side effects, which seem to go away when statin use is stopped: A general sense of feeling unwell, sore throat, headache, digestive issues, peripheral neuropathy.

Several doctors and scientists disagree with using statins with elderly patients (those over 60 years of age) disagreeing with the cholesterol hypothesis that high LDL-C levels cause deposits of plaque, lipids and calcium in the arteries. Their findings are stated in a paper in British Medical Journey Journals (BMJ). You can read the entire study at: https://bmjopen.bmj.com/content/6/6/e010401

I have included a conclusion below.

Lack of an association or an inverse association between low-density-lipoprotein cholesterol and mortality in the elderly: a systematic review

Uffe Ravnskov, David M Diamond, Rokura Hama, Tomohito Hamazaki, Björn Hammarskjöld, Niamh Hynes, Malcolm Kendrick, Peter H Langsjoen, Aseem Malhotra, Luca Mascitelli, Kilmer S McCully, Yoichi Ogushi, Harumi Okuyama, Paul J Rosch, Tore Schersten, Sherif Sultan, Ralf Sundberg

Conclusions
High LDL-C is inversely associated with mortality in most people over 60 years. This finding is inconsistent with the cholesterol hypothesis (ie, that cholesterol, particularly LDL-C, is inherently atherogenic). Since elderly people with high LDL-C live as long or longer than those with low LDL-C, our analysis provides reason to question the validity of the cholesterol hypothesis. Moreover, our study provides the rationale for a re-evaluation of guidelines recommending pharmacological reduction of LDL-C in the elderly as a component of cardiovascular disease prevention strategies.

https://bmjopen.bmj.com/content/6/6/e010401.full?sid=cfb00014-f0a8-407d-ae71-a3278160ca49

see also

https://bmcgeriatr.biomedcentral.com/articles/10.1186/s12877-017-0685-z

Samuel T. Henderson in an article named: *Ketone bodies as a therapeutic for Alzheimer's disease* makes the following observations:

1. Early feature of AD is region-specific declines in glucose metabolism.

2. Inhibition of glucose metabolism can adversely affect brain function

3. A promising approach to this issue is supplementing glucose with keytones

4. Use a diet of high-fat, low-carbohydrate, low-protein to create keytones

5. The benefit comes from the ketone's ability to increase mitochondrial efficiency and supplement the brain's normal reliance on glucose.

See also *The Alzheimer's Antidote: Using a Low-Carib, High-Fat Diet to Fight Alzheimer's Disease, Memory Loss, and Cognitive Decline* by Amy Berger and Dr. David Perlmutter MD. and *The End of Alzheimer's: The First Program to Prevent and Reverse Cognitive Decline* by Dale Bredesen, M.D.

From the US National Library of Medicine National Institutes of Health

A hypothesis out-of-date. the diet-heart idea

Abstract:

An almost endless number of observations and experiments have effectively falsified the hypothesis that dietary cholesterol and fats, and a high cholesterol level play a role in the causation of atherosclerosis and cardiovascular disease. The hypothesis is maintained because allegedly supportive, but insignificant findings, are inflated, and because most contradictory results are misinterpreted, misquoted or ignored.

- https://www.ncbi.nlm.nih.gov/pubmed/12507667

Statins stimulate atherosclerosis and heart failure: pharmacological mechanisms.

Abstract:

In contrast to the current belief that cholesterol reduction with statins decreases atherosclerosis, we present a perspective that statins may be causative in coronary artery calcification and can function as mitochondrial toxins that impair muscle function in the heart and blood vessels through the depletion of coenzyme Q10 and 'heme A', and thereby ATP generation. Statins inhibit the synthesis of vitamin K2, the cofactor for matrix Gla-protein activation, which in turn protects arteries from calcification. Statins inhibit the biosynthesis of selenium containing proteins, one of which is glutathione peroxidase serving to suppress peroxidative stress. An impairment of selenoprotein biosynthesis may be a factor in congestive heart failure, reminiscent of the dilated cardiomyopathies seen with selenium deficiency. Thus, the epidemic of heart failure and atherosclerosis that plagues the modern world may paradoxically be aggravated by the pervasive use of statin drugs. We propose that current statin treatment guidelines be critically reevaluated.

- https://www.ncbi.nlm.nih.gov/pubmed/25655639

Dr. Brownstein warns that the use of statin drugs may:

- Weaken your heart
- Weaken your muscles
- Disrupt your hormone production
- Cause fatigue
- Reduce your sex drive

And it gets even worse, because statins also:

- Put you at risk for brain disorders, including dementia, memory loss, Parkinson's, and ALS (Lou Gehrig's disease)
- Cause kidney and liver problems
- Increase your risk for diabetes and cancer

Dr. David Brownstein is a board-certified family physician and one of the foremost practitioners of holistic medicine in the U.S. He is medical director of the Center for Holistic Medicine in Michigan.

You are not aware of the activity that goes in your body 24 hours a day! It is truly amazing, when you begin to realize everything that is going on in the body and all of that without your direct involvement. You breathe without ever thinking about it. Blood is pumped, oxygen is delivered and CO_2 is removed. The body's operating system attempts to keep everything in balance, such as, blood sugar, body temperature and many other systems critical to life. Invaders are attacked and eliminated. Cells are dying and being replaced. Energy is being produced and information is flowing through a huge network of nerves at a speed we can not imagine. There are thousands of these functions going on 24 hours a day and you don't even know it. All of this activity is happening on a scale so small it is difficult to imagine! You're never aware of it because it happens automatically, like a computer program that is always running. It takes design and information to make it all work. Working virtually without fail (until we stop following the design, adding stress and foreign substances not designed to keep us healthy).

"Endocrine system: Group of ductless glands that secrete hormones necessary for normal growth and development, reproduction, and homeostasis."

– https://sentencedict.com/homeostasis.html

VI

HOMEOSTASIS AND HORMONES

Your body works best when systems are kept within a very small range of tolerances or set points. There are sensors, which relay messages to different glands, which in turn send messages to different parts of the body, to take some action to bring the body back into balance.

Homeostasis, from the Greek meaning "same" and "steady." Because things change in the environment in which we live, the body must have a way to keep systems in balance, like body temperature. One amazing aspect of the human body is its ability to maintain homeostasis. Homeostasis maintains optimal health through multiple feedback systems. These systems are constantly monitoring, evaluating and reevaluating to maintain balance. Without this function, the body would certainly die.

Evolution makes no sense, for the simple reason that undirected chance, natural selection and the idea of adapting can never explain how feedback systems could develop on their own, or how they would know (information) what the optimal levels would be. Take, for instance, the regulation of body temperature. How would undirected chance know that the body needs to maintain a certain temperature? How would it know what the optimal temperature should be? Natural selection would not be any help. There must be something (or someone... a Creator, for instance) that originally designed the entire package. He knew the body's optional temperature had to be near 98.6. There is nothing in nature which could stipulate this on its own. Natural selection would be no help because, for the body to live; all of these feedback systems and regulators have to exist at once. If the body cannot maintain homeostasis in all of its systems, it would soon, overheat, dry up, or any one of the multitudes of critical functions it must have to continue unabated.

Why do we sweat? When you exert yourself to a certain point, you begin to sweat. This is homeostasis at work attempting to maintain temperature. Signals are sent to the appropriate locations, and water is released and the skin is cooled as the water evaporates. When homeostasis is reached, the sweating stops. How did it know to stop sweating? If we did not stop sweating, we would dehydrate and die. That is why it is important to rehydrate after you have been sweating. Unfortunately, it is not only water that you lose but other things as well. Undirected change cannot account for sweating. Natural selection would never have time to work, because the entity would die before it could select the trait. There are a multitude of these systems in the body, working to maintain your health. It is when these systems break down that trouble begins.

The diagram (figure 1a) is an oversimplified example of how the body maintains homeostasis. It is a program that runs to keep things in balance. The body has a thermostat, which will turn on the heat when it gets cold and turn on the air conditioner when it gets too hot. Temperature is just one of the multitudes of systems that must be controlled.

Armed with "INFORMATION" a program could be designed that would maintain homeostasis. However, knowledge of all working parts would be required for it to work properly. By changing one aspect of your body's system without knowing how it will affect other parts is a recipe for disaster. Therefore, this is an all-or-nothing proposition. It requires a designed operating system that is aware of all of its parts and how they interrelate. Hormones are used to maintain homeostasis. For our purposes in this book, we will concentrate on hormones that have to do with nutritional health: insulin, leptin, ghrelin, adiponectin, resistin, interleukin, apelin, tumor necrosis factor, glucagon, and estrogen.

What is a hormone? Hormones are like a switch when it reaches a cell the hormone receptor tells the cell to take a specific action.

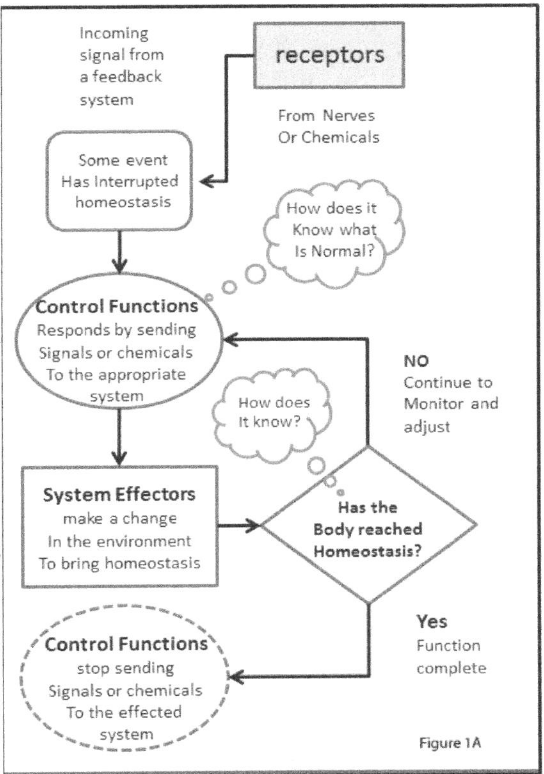

Insulin is an anabolism for storing glucose in the cell which can be used to generate energy in the mitochondria. Insulin is a fat storing hormone produced in the pancreas by the beta cells. Studies have shown that adding insulin will actually cause you to gain fat!

Figure 1A

Maintaining Homeostasis

Insulin blocks the production of leptin. Leptin is a hormone that tells your brain that you are full. The more insulin in the blood stream the hungrier you feel. The hungrier you feel the more you eat, now your brain tells the body you have reached a starvation level and starts storing the glucose as fat!

When cells are overwhelmed by increased insulin levels, the cells become insensitive to the action of the hormone, and glucose is not allowed to enter the cell and remains in the blood stream resulting in a high blood-sugar level. I think about my first trip to New York City. All night long there was sirens, traffic and noise. After a period of time, my mind filtered out the irritating noise similarly to the way cells stop glucose from entering.

Increased sugar in the blood and insulin resistance is the cause of many of the health issues we have today: obesity, diabetes, hypertension, heart disease and others. It has been said the insulin resistance is also responsible for some cancers and brain disorders like Alzheimer.

The HbA1c blood test reveals a blood-sugar level over a period of three months. A reading of over 5.7 will indicate insulin resistance.

Leptin
Visfatin
Adiponectin
Apelin
ADIPOSE TISSUE
Resistin
Estrogen
Tumor necrosis factor
Interleukins

Glucagon is a catabolism which is used to burn fat. This hormone is produced in the pancreas by the alpha cells.

Insulin is a hormone, a trigger for the cell to accept glucose and glucagon is a hormone trigger to burn fat.

LEPTIN is a hormone made by adipose (fat) cells to indicate that you have enough food.

Failure in Homeostasis: Diabetes

The pancreas is what controls blood sugar. When it is too low, the pancreas releases glucose to maintain homeostasis. When it is too high, the liver synthesizes and stores it. Glucose homeostasis is governed by the interplay of insulin, glucagon, amylin, and incretin hormones.

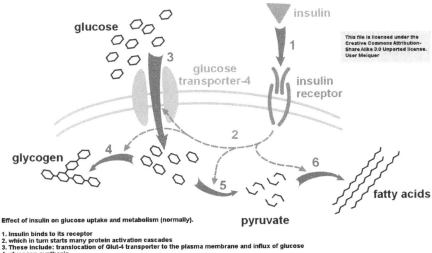

Effect of insulin on glucose uptake and metabolism (normally).

1. Insulin binds to its receptor
2. which in turn starts many protein activation cascades
3. These include: translocation of Glut-4 transporter to the plasma membrane and influx of glucose
4. glycogen synthesis
5. glycolysis
6. and fatty acid synthesis

We are all familiar with insulin and glucagon. Insulin is sent out from the pancreas to tell cells to accept glucose from the blood stream. If blood sugar is still too high, insulin will bind to the liver and cause it to take in glucose. Glucose is a monomer, meaning a single unit. The glucose molecules come together in the liver to form glycogen, a polymer, made up of several glucose molecules.

When blood sugar levels fall, the pancreas excretes the hormone glucagon, which binds to the liver and the liver converts the stored glycogen molecules back into glucose and releases it into the bloodstream.

Amylin was first discovered in 1987 and was found to help the regulation of glycemic levels in the blood. Amylin is released with insulin in the b-cells. Here is how amylin works:

> The overall effect is to slow the rate of appearance (Ra) of glucose in the blood after eating; this is accomplished via coordinate slowing down gastric emptying, inhibition of

digestive secretion [gastric acid, pancreatic enzymes, and bile ejection], and a resulting reduction in food intake. - Ratner RE, Dickey R, Fineman M, Maggs DG, Shen L, Strobel SA, Weyer C, Kolterman OG; Dickey; Fineman; Maggs; Shen; Strobel; Weyer; Kolterman (2004). *"Amylin replacement with pramlintide as an adjunct to insulin therapy improves long-term glycaemic and weight control in Type 1 diabetes mellitus: a 1-year, randomized controlled trial"*.

In the case of type II diabetes (90% of cases), the issue can be a result of many factors; the pancreas does not create enough b-cells (used to store and release insulin); the insulin receptor on the cells become insensitive to insulin signaling, resulting in hyperglycemia (an increase in circulating glucose in the blood). The onset of type II diabetes occurs when the insulin receptor on the cell fails to respond. Things that cause this issue are, being obese, lack of exercise, genetic predisposition and eating habits.

Why is blood sugar regulation so important? If the blood sugar in the blood gets too low, the production of energy in the form of ATP slows down or stops. This, if not corrected will result in death or a coma. If blood sugar is too high, water in the cells move to the high concentration of glucose in the blood, resulting in reduced water in the cells. If the blood-glucose level is not reduced, you become thirsty or in extreme cases dehydrated. Regular sodas are overly concentrated with sugar, since this raises the sugar in the blood, water is extracted from cells. This is why sodas never quench your thirst, but make you thirstier. The tendency is then to drink more. Good for the soda manufacturers; not so good for us...

Our bodies were designed to operate in a specific way, if we overwhelm it with overly processed foods and chemicals (see endocrine disruptors later in this chapter) and a lack of movement, the result is poor health. To blame God for death and disease is pointing the finger in the wrong direction. It is sin, greed and the lack of human understanding that causes most of our issues, just like soda companies who put enormous amounts of sodium and sugar in their products to increase thirst and the need to drink another "Mega Soda."

Calcium Homeostasis

There are two hormones that regulate calcium homeostasis; parathyroid hormone and calcitonin. When calcium is low (Where did the information come from that determines what is an optimal level of calcium?) the parathyroid gland sends a hormone signal to the bones to release calcium in the blood to be used by cells in the body. In the case where calcium is perceived to be too high, calcitonin is released to slow the release of calcium. Calcitonin is produced by the c-cells in the thyroid gland.

When too much calcium has released a condition known as hypercalcemia occurs. This condition, if not corrected by calcitonin, can cause kidney stones, organ damage and osteoporosis because too much calcium is being released from the bones.

Hypocalcemia is caused when there is not enough calcium in the blood and cells. This condition can also cause osteoporosis, muscle spasms and osteomalacia, which is the softening of bones. In children, it is known as rickets. Because of the lack of vitamin D and poor absorption of calcium this condition can cause to serve deformation. In adults, it causes muscle weakness, various body pains and fragile bones.

Fight or Flight:

This is not considered homeostasis in a strict sense, but it is related to it as self-preservation. There are multiple chemical reactions and signals sent through the body by nerves and the blood stream. All of these reactions take place in an extremely short time. I have a very high-level flow chart that explains what happens when we are stressed or scared. This is not a detailed example, as there are many other chemical reactions that take place.

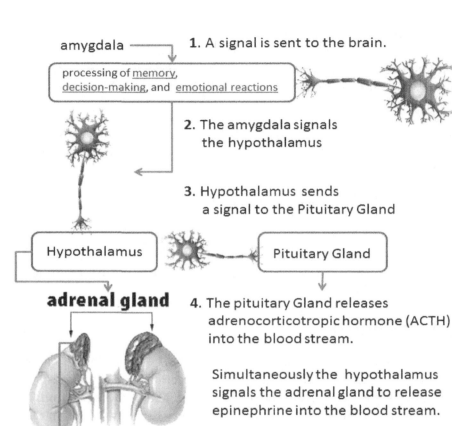

amygdala ——— **1.** A signal is sent to the brain.

processing of <u>memory</u>, <u>decision-making</u>, and <u>emotional reactions</u>

2. The amygdala signals the hypothalamus

3. Hypothalamus sends a signal to the Pituitary Gland

Hypothalamus

Pituitary Gland

adrenal gland

4. The pituitary Gland releases adrenocorticotropic hormone (ACTH) into the blood stream.

Simultaneously the hypothalamus signals the adrenal gland to release epinephrine into the blood stream.

Kidneys

5. The receptor on the adrenal gland causes the G protein complex to activate, this stimulates adenylate cyclase to convert into cAMP.

6. Several chemical reactions take place and the final result is **cortisol** which will leave the cell and enter the blood stream..

CORTISOL

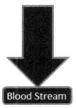

7. The release of **cortisol** into the blood stream
   Causes several reactions in the body:

   - Increase in blood pressure
   - Increase in blood sugar levels
   - Suppression of the immune system

8. Epinephrine which was released earlier on, start to effect other cells in the body.

The signal takes the liver through several different chemical reactions,to create a store of glucose, which is released into the blood stream. This glucose provides energy for the muscles.

Epinephrine

On the Skin, it binds to a receptor which causes the hair to stand up. On the surface, it causes the sweat gland to release sweat.

In the lungs, epinephrine causes the muscle cells to relax so there is an increase in respiration.

In the heart, epinephrine stimulates the cells so they beat faster, causing an increase in signaling through out the body.

Acid-base homeostasis (pH): potential hydrogen or the

concentration of hydrogen ions in the blood.

It is measured logarithmically and reveals how acidic or alkaline an aqueous solution is. The measurement of pH is logarithmic, 6 is ten times more acidic than 7.

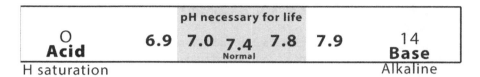

What you eat affects your pH level; meat, eggs, dairy, beans, nuts and seeds are more acidic, where fruits and vegetables are typically more alkaline.

You normally have a pH of about 7.4 in the blood. You can live when pH reaches a level as high as 7.8 or as low as 7.0, beyond that, enzymes and electric systems don't operate correctly, and eventually the body will shut down. The more acidic," the hotter" things are, the faster they respond. The more alkaline the body, "the colder" things get the slower they react. When the body cools, electrical reactions become more resistance, and nerve impulses slow down. Enzymes and proteins have an optimal pH range, once outside they become inactive or denatured.

While writing this book, I could not find anyone who knew all the mechanisms that keep the blood pH at 7.4. The kidneys can adjust states of excess but not deficiency and the kidneys, and the lungs work together to buffer the pH level in the blood.

Minerals are critical for optimal health; pH balance affects the assimilation of minerals. The deficiency of minerals is known to be associated with many diseases: Cancer, Arthritis, Diabetes, Anorexia, Hypertension.

Exercise

During exercise, oxygen is used to convert glucose into energy (ATP), CO_2 and $H+$ are the result of the energy process. This is then, carried out of the muscle, by the blood, this causes the pH level to drop. Because of the wonderful design of our bodies, we have buffers. Kidneys will remove excess chemicals from the blood, if the kidneys can not remove the chemicals fast enough the result is metabolic acidosis. This is where the lungs play their part in removing excess CO_2 through heavy breathing. If the lungs cannot remove enough CO_2 the result is respiratory acidosis.

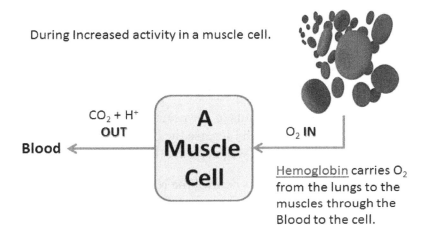

During Increased activity in a muscle cell.

$CO_2 + H^+$
OUT

Blood

A Muscle Cell

O_2 IN

Hemoglobin carries O_2 from the lungs to the muscles through the Blood to the cell.

Different parts of the body have different pH levels depending on its function. Gastric acid is generally around 1; so digestive system can "digest" foods. The stomach's pH is between 4 and 6.5; the lower part of the stomach is very acidic 1.5 to 4. When the food enters the small intestine, the pH is more alkaline with a pH of 7 to 8.5. This is where the absorption of nutrients occurs, the waste product is sent to the colon, which is again very acidic with a pH of 4 to 7.

If your body is not slightly alkaline, the body cannot heal itself. If your pH is not balanced you will not be able to assimilate nutrients effectively.

Blood Pressure Homeostasis:

Low blood pressure is called hypotension and can be caused by things like dehydration and loss blood from a major cut. Hypotension, if not corrected, can cause fainting or worse, kidney failure. Hypertension occurs when the blood pressure is too high and can ultimately, if not brought into balance, cause a stroke.

There are two hormones which affect the cardiovascular system, ADH (anti-diuretic hormone - stimulates contraction of arteries and capillaries) and epinephrine (known as adrenaline).

The baroreceptor (baro means pressure) found in the carotid sinuses (blood which is going to the brain) and the aortic arch (blood going to the body) are receptors. These receptors communicate to the brain changes in **the stretch,** in the veins. The brain remembers what your normal set point is, say 120/80 because of the number of action potentials it receives through the central nervous system. If that number goes up, the brain knows that blood pressure is above normal. If the number of action potentials goes down, then the brain knows that blood pressure is dropping.

There are two nervous system inputs to the heart, sympathetic input and parasympathetic. Sympathetic will increase the heart rate pumping more blood and parasympathetic input will decrease the rate.

Additionally, endothelial receptors control the restriction of blood vessels. These receptors are found in the smooth muscle tissue of blood vessels. Endothelins attempt to maintain a balance between vasoconstriction (constriction) and vasodilation. (dilation) of blood vessels.

The human body is an extremely complex machine. Hormones and feedback systems attempt to keep us in balance through homeostasis. However, problems begin when we overwhelm the system with chemicals, stress, inappropriate diets and other factors. When medical professionals try to remedy the issues with drugs and invasive procedures the problem will often get worse. It is critical that we know *what caused the issue* if we are to reverse the problem in the long run. This I am afraid is usually not the case.

The constant conditions which are maintained in the body might be termed equilibria. That word, however, has come to have fairly exact meaning as applied to relatively simple physico-chemical states, in closed systems, where known forces are balanced. The coordinated physiological processes which maintain most of the steady states in the organism are so complex and so peculiar to living beings—involving, as they may, the brain and nerves, the heart, lungs, kidneys and spleen, all working cooperatively—that I have suggested a special designation for these states, homeostasis. The word does not imply something set and immobile, a stagnation. It means a condition—a condition which may vary, but which is relatively constant.

— Walter Bradford Cannon *In The Wisdom of the Body* (1932), 24.

"If only a small fraction of what is already known about the effects of sugar were to be revealed in relation to any other material used as a food additive, that material would promptly be banned. "

- Dr. John Yudkin - *Sugar - Pure White and Deadly.*

VII

SUGAR
Pure, White and Deadly

Pure White and Deadly is the title of a book written by Dr. John Yudkin in 1972. His nemesis was the infamous Ancel Keys. Keys was being paid by the sugar industry. Keys pushed back on everything Yudkin brought forth. There are many researchers and medical professionals who are now pushing back against the lie about sugar. Yes, I said LIE because that is what it has been and still is today. ***FOLLOW THE MONEY!***

"...Directors of a large food-manufacturing firm (:)...At one extreme (: one) said it was not his job to protect people from themselves; he was not forcing people to eat his products, and if they chose to do so at the risk of harming themselves, it was of their own free choice." - Dr. John Yudkin - *Sugar - Pure White and Deadly.*

During Yudkin's time (the 1970s) the sugar industry had this in their advertising:

'Willpower fans, the search is over! And guess where it's at? In sugar! Sugar works faster than any other food to turn your appetite down, turn energy up. Spoil your appetite with sugar, and you could come up with willpower. Sugar - only 18 calories per teaspoon, and it's all energy.'

Think about it, from your experience, if you have drunk any of the sugar laden sodas, does anything in the ad ring true? NO, I would say it is full of miss-characterizations. You most likely would never see an ad like that today. Does it turn down your appetite? No, from my experience, if anything because of the sugar and sodium you will NOT be satisfied and will require more. Will it turn your energy up? Yes, very temporarily, but it will cause a crash in energy later, unless you keep drinking or eating more sugar. The reason for this crash is because carbohydrates are used immediately. The deception comes when they say, "only 18 calories" look at the actual number of calories in a can of coke, it is 140 and 50 mg of sodium! The super size soda at the local convenience has 312 calories and 91 mg of sodium.

Today, our foods are full of excess sugar. Just look at virtually any packaged food. You will find added sugars. Research tells us that 80% of food items in a store will have added sugar. Just remember to multiply the sugar grams by the total servings in the package, another trick to hide the total amount of sugar in a packaged food.

The following is a list of sugars you may encounter in your food:

agave nectar	barley malt	blackstrap molasses
brown rice syrup sugar	brown sugar	coconut
cane sugar	corn syrup	date sugar
dextrin	diastatic malt	dextrose
ethyl maltol	florida crystals	fructose
fruit juice	glucose	golden syrup
high-fructose corn syrup	honey	lactose
levulose	maltodextrin	muscovado
maltose	maple sugar	molasses
nonfat dry milk	palm sugar	panocha
sorgum syurp	sorbitol	saccharose
skimmed milk	powder sorghum	sucrose
treacle	turbinado	

Yudkin points out the falacy of their propaganda. Leading the charge today is Dr. Robert Lustig M.D. and Kristen Kerns DDS and probably others.

In the vein of "Supersize Me", Damon Gameau becomes a human guinea-pig when he puts himself through a grueling 6 week diet consuming the equivalent of 40 teaspoons of sugar a day... the average daily amount consumed by teenagers! This bold, colorful and entertaining film explores all things "sweet" and exposes the damage that fructose (processed sugar) is doing to a generation of addicts.

- *That Sugar Film*

> "Sugar can act like poison in high doses—and the amount in our diets has gone beyond toxic," - Robert Lustig, M.D.,

In Nicole Avena's book, *Why Diets Fail: Because You're addicted to Sugar,* she says about the added sugar in our foods: "Repeated spikes can desensitize that center, which could release less and less dopamine, leaving you needing more and more sugar to score a rush. These are the same brain patterns you see during drug addiction." And "We see brain changes that lead to lethargy, anxiety, and irritability, And also changes that produce fierce cravings."

Fructose

Fructose is found in fruits and vegetables in varying amounts. Table sugar is 50 percent glucose and 50% fructose. Glucose can be delivered to energy throughout the body. However, fructose sugar is delivered directly to the liver for processing. If the liver is overwhelmed continuously by the flood of fructose, the process of lipogenesis kicks in, and you end up with fatty liver disease. The overabundance of fructose has the tendency to lower the "good" cholesterol HDL increasing the potential for multiple metabolic syndromes.

High-fructose corn syrup (HFCS) is a combination of glucose and fructose. HFCS is used because it is very sweet, several times sweeter than sucrose and lower in cost than other sugars. It is generally said that fructose comes from fruit, but that is not the case. Where most sugars can be metabolized in the cell, fructose must be metabolized in the liver. The liver then converts the fructose to glucose and fat. When high amounts of fructose are consumed over time the liver becomes overwhelmed and the result is known as non-alcoholic fatty liver (NAFL - Hepatic Steatosis). What this implies is that **fructose is as damaging as alcohol,** and it has the same effects on the liver as alcohol (ethanol) a known toxin.

HFCS comes in several different strengths HFCS-90, which is 90% fructose, HFCS-55, which is 55% fructose and 42 % glucose and other combinations. HFCS-55 is close to table sugar in its chemical makeup and is deemed as "safe." However, both will have negative outcomes if used in excess. Check the label to see if the product you are buying has excess sugar. You will be surprised to find out how many products, even those that are advertised as healthy. HFCS is said to come from GMO (genetically modified organism) corn.

Fructose causes a reaction in the body that creates AGEs (advanced glycation end-products); the AGEs cause oxidative damage in the cells and will lead to inflammation and therefore, other chronic diseases. Fructose can also be traced back to the cause of dyslipidemia (excess lipids [fat] in the blood).

Fructose also affects leptin, a hormone that tells the brain that you have eaten enough. If that hormone is not activated, you will continue to eat even though you would have normally stopped. This is another way that fructose causes weight gain.

Obesity is a major epidemic, but its causes are still unclear. In this article, we investigate the relation between the intake of high-fructose corn syrup (HFCS) and the development of obesity. Using the US Department of Agriculture food consumption tables from 1967 to 2000 we find that the consumption of HFCS increased > 1000% between 1970 and 1990. HFCS now represents > 40% of caloric sweeteners added to foods and beverages and is the sole caloric sweetener in soft drinks in the United States

The American Journal of Clinical Nutrition, Volume 79, Issue 4, April 2004, Pages 537–543, https://doi.org/10.1093/ajcn/79.4.537

Fructose and Gout

Gout occurs when the body does not rid itself of excess uric acid. Why? Kidney damage caused by high insulin and high glucose which are symptom of insulin resistance. Obesity, type II diabetes, High-Fructose Corn Syrup and Purines like red meat, shellfish and organ meat can also contribute but are not the cause. However, it is the kidney's job to rid the body of excess uric acid.

Diet may be a factor. High intake of dietary purine, high-fructose corn syrup, and table sugar can increase levels of uric acid. -

Angelopoulos, Theodore J.; Lowndes, Joshua; Zukley, Linda; Melanson, Kathleen J.; Nguyen, Von; Huffman, Anik; Rippe, James M. (June 2009). "*The Effect of High-Fructose Corn Syrup Consumption on Triglycerides and Uric Acid*". J. Nutr. 139 (6): 1242S–1245S. doi:10.3945/jn.108.098194. PMID 19403709.

High-fructose diet stimulates hepatic de novo lipogenesis (DNL) and causes hypertriglyceridemia and insulin resistance in rodents. Fructose-induced insulin resistance may be secondary to alterations of lipid metabolism. - US National Library of Medicine National Institutes of Health. *Effect of fructose overfeeding and fish oil administration on hepatic de novo lipogenesis and insulin sensitivity in healthy men.*

RECENT FINDINGS:

There are many recently published epidemiological studies that provide evidence that sugar consumption is associated with metabolic disease. Three recent clinical studies, which investigated the effects of consuming relevant doses of sucrose or high-fructose corn syrup along with ad libitum diets ["as you desire" *where the amount of food is not restricted*], provide evidence that consumption of these sugars increase the risk factors for cardiovascular disease and metabolic syndrome. Mechanistic studies suggest that these effects result from the rapid hepatic metabolism of fructose catalyzed by fructokinase C, which generates substrate for de novo lipogenesis and leads to increased uric acid levels. Recent clinical studies investigating the effects of consuming less sugar, via educational interventions or by substitution of sugar-sweetened beverages for noncalorically sweetened beverages, provide evidence that such strategies have beneficial effects on risk factors for metabolic disease or on BMI in children. - US National Library of Medicine National Institutes of Health.

Adverse metabolic effects of dietary fructose: results from the recent epidemiological, clinical, and mechanistic studies.

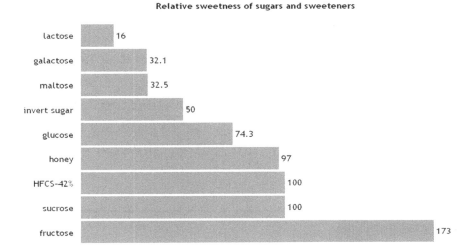

Relative sweetness of sugars and sweeteners

Galactose

Galactose is not as sweet as sucrose. Galactose is found in dairy, avocados and sugar beets.

Sugar and Cancer

The University of Texas at Dallas has found a link between sugar and cancer after they analyzed data from The Cancer Genome Atlas .

Starve cancer by stop feeding it glucose! Cancer cells thrive on sugar but generally do not have receptors for keytone bodies. The enzyme Phosphoinositide 3-kinase is involved in cell growth, survival and other functions at the cellular level.

Lewis Cantley, PhD. (director of the Meyer Cancer Center) said that the PI3K enzyme (Phosphoinositide 3-kinase), which is activated by insulin, drives glucose into a cell. However, cancer cells "hijack" the enzyme feeding the cancer rather than sending it to muscle, the cells or the adipose (fat) tissue.

"What has gone wrong? In other fields, when bridges do not stand, when aircraft do not fly. When machines do not work, **when treatments do not cure**, despite all the conscientious efforts on the part of many persons to make them do so. One begins to question the basic assumptions, principles, theories, and hypotheses that guide one's efforts." — Aurthur Jensen, University of California

"But fear not, there does appear to be one dietary item that can mitigate the damage that sugar does to the brain and promote the biochemistry and the processes that can predispose us to happiness. And perhaps not surprisingly its presence in the diet correlates positively with tryptophan and negatively with sugar. What is this magic chemical? It's omega-3 fatty acids, of all things."

Dr. Robert H. Lustig, The Hacking of the American Mind: Inside the Sugar-Coated Plot to Confuse Pleasure with Happiness

"Rats given sweetened water in experiments find it significantly more pleasurable than cocaine, even when they're addicted to the latter, and more than heroin as well (although the rats find this choice more difficult to make). Addict"

— Gary Taubes, The Case Against Sugar

https://www.ncbi.nlm.nih.gov/pmc/articles/PMC3969361/

Intake of Fruit Juice and Incidence of Type 2 Diabetes: A Systematic Review and Meta-Analysis

Bo Xi, 1 Shuangshuang Li, 1 Zhaolu Liu, 1 Huan Tian, 1 Xiuxiu Yin, 1 Pengcheng Huai, 2 Weihong Tang, 3 Donghao Zhou, 4 , * and Lyn M. Steffen 3 , Olga Y. Gorlova, Editor

Abstract

Background

Several prospective studies have been conducted to examine the relationship between fruit juice intake and risk of incident type 2 diabetes, but results have been mixed. In the present study, we aimed to estimate the association between fruit juice intake and risk of type 2 diabetes.

Methods

PubMed and Embase databases were searched up to December 2013. All prospective cohort studies of fruit juice intake with risk of type 2 diabetes were included. The pooled relative risks (RRs) with 95% confidence intervals (CIs) for highest vs. lowest category of fruit juice intake were estimated using a random-effects model.

Results

A total of four studies (191,686 participants, including 12,375 with type 2 diabetes) investigated the association between sugar-sweetened fruit juice and risk of incident type 2 diabetes, and four studies (137,663 participants and 4,906 cases) investigated the association between 100% fruit juice and risk of incident type 2 diabetes. A higher intake of sugar-sweetened fruit juice was significantly associated with risk of type 2 diabetes (RR=1.28, 95%CI=1.04–1.59, p=0.02), while intake of 100% fruit juice was not associated with risk of developing type 2 diabetes (RR=1.03, 95% CI=0.91–1.18, p=0.62).

"The effects of added sugar intake — higher blood pressure, inflammation, weight gain, diabetes, and fatty liver disease — are all linked to an increased risk for heart attack and stroke," says Dr. Hu.

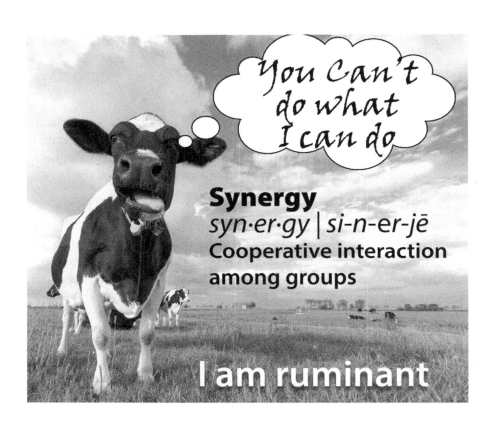

VIII

Ruminants

"It's what's for Dinner"

(an advertising slogan and campaign aimed to promote
the benefits of incorporating beef into a healthy diet.
© Beef Industry Council)

Ruminants do for you what you cannot for yourself. The domestic ruminants are animals like; cows, goats and sheep. Ruminants are characterized by the fact that they have four stomachs and can process grass into human edible meat full of nutrients. These nutrients (from grasses) are not accessible by humans because our digestive system cannot process it like ruminants can. We then have a synergistic relationship with ruminants because they provide us high-quality nutrition by converting vegetation, which is not edible by humans, and turns it into a food source with all the nutrients needed for health.

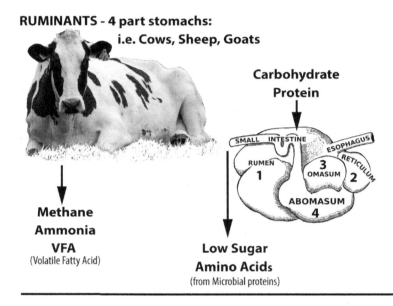

RUMINANTS - 4 part stomachs:
i.e. Cows, Sheep, Goats

Carbohydrate
Protein

SMALL INTESTINE   ESOPHAGUS
RUMEN 3 RETICULUM
1 OMASUM 2
ABOMASUM
4

Methane
Ammonia
VFA
(Volatile Fatty Acid)

Low Sugar
Amino Acids
(from Microbial proteins)

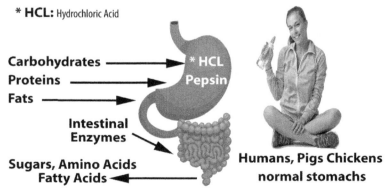

* HCL: Hydrochloric Acid

Carbohydrates ⟶
Proteins ⟶
Fats ⟶

* HCL
Pepsin

Intestinal
Enzymes

Sugars, Amino Acids
Fatty Acids ◀

Humans, Pigs Chickens
normal stomachs

Why we need Ruminates:

> "There's a difference between ingestion and digestion. We are not what we eat, we are what our body does with what we eat and that's a significant difference. And so the fat content of the diet of any ruminant is going to be below 6% fat and yet thanks to this microbial fermentation that converts carbohydrates into fats 70% to 80% of the caloric needs of these animals are coming from fat. Isn't that an amazing trick? Eat carbohydrates and absorb fat. So we should let the ruminants convert the carbs to fat for us instead of us.
>
> - Dr. Peter Ballerstedt - Agronomist

Humans, chickens and pigs have stomachs, which are not capable of digesting grass (we are mono-gastric). Our stomachs are based on digestion using an acid compound. The ruminant's digestion is based on fermentation and bacteria.

The protein and vitamins in vegetation cannot always be utilized by our bodies, and in some cases these plants contain lectins and phytates. Lectins and Phytates are considered anti nutrients and are the cause of "leaky gut syndrome." As the name implies, leaky gut is a state where the lining of the intestine has "holes." These holes allow undigested food, toxins and bacteria to enter the tissues outside of the intestine. This leaking of materials causes a number of chronic diseases; Crohn's, celiac disease and irritable bowl syndrome, autoimmune diseases, and a potential for other maladies. Some turn to soy as a source of protein. The issues with soy are many.

1. The phytoestrogens in soy are similar to the hormone estrogen and will interfere with normal hormone metabolism. This can result in breast cancer, endometriosis, male infertility and in rare cases gynecomastia (man breasts).

2. Upwards of 80% of soybeans production in the US are GMOs.

3. It can interfere with normal thyroid function

157

Animal foods are the best most available source of vitamin B_{12}. Highest concentrations come from organ meats from lamb, beef, mackerel and crab. Symptoms of B_{12} deficiency are: fatigue, depression, poor memory, balance issues and lethargy.

> "Ruminants increase the human-edible food supply! At least half of their feed cannot be eaten by humans."
>
> - Dr. Peter Ballerstedt - Agronomist

We have a synergistic relationship with ruminants. Dr. Ballerstedt gives us an essential macro-nutrient comparison.

Humans Need:	Macro-nutient	Ruminants Need:
Yes-------------	Amino Acids	No
Yes------------	Fatty Acids	No
No	Carbohydrates---------	**Yes**

Dr. Ballerstedt lists several benefits of ruminants to humans: From Peter J Soest, 1982: *The nutricianal Ecology of the Ruminant*

- They convert carbohydrates into human digestible fat

- They convert plant protein into animal protein

- They provide B_{12} and other vitamins

- They increase the availability of essential minerals

- They maintain the health of grassland ecosystems

- They Recycle nutrients and build soil health

- They provide byproducts like leather

Ruminant digestive system

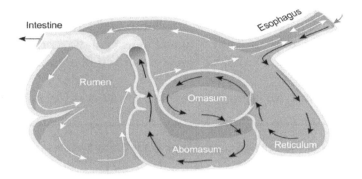

How does the ruminant system work?

1. Grass is consumed and crushed
2. The content is moved to the rumen
3. The content is mixed with microorganisms whereby it breaks down cellulose and other compounds to simple sugars by fermentation.
4. This mixture is converted to acetic acid and butyric acid and absorbed in the blood for energy. This fermentation creates methane gas.
5. Rumen bacteria combine the inorganic nitrogen to make proteins at the same time create B-complex and K vitamins. The result is Volatile Fatty Acids (VFAs) a high quality nutrient for the ruminant animal.
6. The cud is regurgitated to the reticulum for further processing then moved back to the mouth where it is chewed again.
7. The result is moved to the 3rd chamber the omasum where water is absorbed and the digestive enzyme lysozyme breaks down the bacteria to release nutrients.
8. The content is then passed to the abomasum where digestive enzymes to extract protein from plant cells.
9. Then it passes to the small intestine for final processing.

The ruminant has the ability to breakdown cellulose and convert it to fat. This is why a cow can get so large. You can be a vegetarian if you want to, although, there are nutritional issues if you eat that way. We are designed to eat meat and can eat fruits and vegetables; we are omnivores [omnis - all, and vora - to eat or devour]. The herbivores have a much longer digestive system and other facilities to digest the cellulose in plant material. Our digestive system is more like the carnivores. We have digestive enzymes where herbivores have microbes. We are "hind gut" fermenters meaning we ferment in the colon. We are not designed to ferment fiber. The amount of SCFAs (short chain fatty acids) we can absorb from fiber is less than 10%.

However scientists have recently reclassified humans as Cucinivores.

> **Humans as Cucinivores: Comparisons With Other Species**
> John B Furness, David M Bravo
>
> The human digestive system is suited to a processed food diet because of its smaller volume, notably smaller colonic volume, relative to the intestines of other species, and because of differences from other primates in dentition and facial muscles that result in lower bite strength. There is no known group of humans which does not consume cooked foods, and the modern diet is dominated by processed foods. We conclude that humans are well adapted as consumers of processed, including cooked, foods.
>
> https://pubmed.ncbi.nlm.nih.gov/26123626/

We get a lot of essential (meaning not made in the body) amino acids from meat that are not found in plants. There are nine essential amino acids: histidine, leucine, lycine, isoleucine, methionine, phenylalanine, threonine, tryptophan, valine. Meat is a rich source of B vitamins: niacin, folic acid, thiamine, biotin, pantothenic acid, vitamin B12, and vitamin B6 each has a purpose in keeping us healthy.

A major problem with many of the epidemiological studies is that it requires the participant to remember what they ate over a long period of time. Something like "how many apples did you eat last year". I don't know about you, but I could not accurately respond to that question. Yet, the results of these studies often use this as proof of their hypothesis.

"The biggest problem is that the vast majority of studies are not experimental, randomized designs. Simply by observing what people eat—or even worse, what they recall they ate—and trying to link this to disease outcomes is moreover a waste of effort. These studies need to be largely abandoned. We've wasted enough resources and caused enough confusion." —Professor John Ioannidis, MD, 2018"

"For most of human history, browsers and grazers haven't been in competition with humans. They ate what we couldn't eat—cellulose— and turned it into what we could—protein and fat. Grain will dramatically increase the growth rate of beef cattle (there's a reason for the expression "cornfed") and the milk production of dairy cows. It will also kill them. The delicate bacterial balance of a cow's rumen will go acid and turn septic. Chickens get fatty liver disease if fed grain exclusively, and they don't need any grain to survive. Sheep and goats, also ruminants, should really never touch the stuff."

- Lierre Keith - *The Vegetarian Myth: Food, Justice and Sustainability*

The Carnivore Diet With Intermittent Fasting by Michael D. Kaiser Special Edition - Two Books Intermittent Fasting The science is "in" on the many methods of Intermittent Fasting. The health benefits and metabolic benefits are significant and proven many times over through clinical trials; Anti-aging, fat loss, weight loss, reduced hunger, clarity and much more. The newest rage in the low carb community is the Carnivore Diet. People are are reporting tremendously beneficial results in digestion, energy and fat loss/weight loss. Completely contradictory to what doctors have been preaching for years about what comprises a "healthy" diet. Book One: The Carnivore Diet"Eat meat only - Get lean and healthy". Book Two: Intermittent Fasting Weight Loss – Health Benefits – End Cravings and Dieting – Increased Energy " quoted from the book on Amazon.com

"Lectins, in particular, block absorption of calcium, iron, phosphorus, and zinc — essential minerals you need "

Are anti-nutrients harmful? The Nutrition Source,
T.H. Chan School of Public Health, Harvard University. Accessed 22 Mar 2019.

IX

REVENGE
Of The
Plant Empire

Lectins

Plants are not always helpless against invaders who would eat them. There is a chemical that is very dangerous contained in and on plants known as lectins. I am NOT saying that you should not eat plants that have lectins, only that you should *cook them appropriately*.

Sources of Lectins:

Soy beans	kidney beans	navy beans
pinto beans	lima Bbeans	fava beans
wax beans	castor beans	jack beans
string beans	Sweet peas	green peas
cow peas	horse grams	barley
corn	rice	wheat
wheat germ	tomatoes	potatoes
sweet potatoes	zucchini	carrots
rhubarb	beets	mushrooms
asparagus	turnips	cucumbers
pumpkin	sweet peppers	radishes
oranges	lemons	grapefrui
blackberries	raspberries	strawberries.
pomegranate	grapes	cherries
quinces	apples	watermelon
banana	papaya	plums
currants	Walnuts	hazelnuts
peanuts	sunflower seeds	sesame seeds
coconut	chocolate	coffee
caraway	nutmeg	peppermint
marjoram	garlic	egg plant

Cornell University: Plant Lectins

Kidney beans, if eaten raw cause vomiting, and diarrhea. Lectins are proteins that can bind to carbohydrates (glyca-binding protein). The lectins that bind to our cells can damage the lining of our guts. Lectins are considered as pro inflammatory, immunotoxic, neurotoxic and cytotoxic (see appendix A glossary of terms). This inflammatory process causes the endothelia cells (the squamous cells that line the interior of blood vessels and the lymphatic vessels) to come loose causing "leaky gut" (see appendix B). Lectins can also cause apoptosis of cells. Because we cannot digest lectins, the body sees them as foreign invaders and sets off an inflammatory response. C-reactive protein (CRP) is the liver's response to inflammation.

Lectins are referred to as anti-nutrients. Eating too many foods containing lectins has been known to cause rheumatoid arthritis and celiac disease.

Lectins when bound to a cell can give the incorrect instructions, or it can block the binding of hormones essential for appropriate cell function.

Effects of wheat germ agglutinin on insulin binding and insulin sensitivity of fat cells.

Abstract

The plant lectin (wheat germ agglutinin, WGA) produces several alterations in the ability of fat cells to bind and respond to insulin. Although WGA markedly stimulated glucose oxidation, it caused only a modest stimulation of glucose transport. WGA (0.25-20 micrograms/ml) increased the binding of insulin by adipocytes, apparently by increasing the binding affinity of the insulin receptor. With low WGA concentrations (0.25-2.5 micrograms/ml), the elevation in binding was accompanied by an increase in the sensitivity of the adipocytes to insulin stimulation of glucose transport.

PMID: 6989266 DOI: 10.1152/ajpendo.1980.238.3.E267 - https://www.ncbi.nlm.nih.gov/pubmed/6989266

One of the reasons that people experience joint pain is that lectins will bind to glucosamine a polysaccharide (also known as a glycan) found in the joints and interferes with normal function.

Lectins are also known to promote leptin resistance. Leptin is a hormone that lets your brain realize that you are full and to stop eating. Without that chemical response you continue to eat beyond what you need. The result is the storage of fat.

"Stories of lectin poisoning are not especially rare. In 'The Independent' (*The Independent* September 15, 2008) the food writer Vicky Jones describes a dinner party in which she used Greek butter beans in a dish without boiling them first. Soon everyone was violently ill. It came on so quickly that before they could consider going to the emergency room, death seemed preferable to [trekking to the] hospital. Jones recovered fully, as most lectin-poisoned people do." - *The Atlantic* April 24, 2017

Lectins can also induce an insulin response. As we have already indicated, insulin is what causes fat to be stored in the adipose cells. According to a study :

Bound lectins that mimic insulin produce persistent insulin-like activities

Abstract:

"Short preincubation of rat adipocytes with wheat germ agglutinin, followed by removal of unbound lectin, resulted in persistent activation of lipogenesis, which lasted at least 3h. The bound lectin also inhibited lipolysis initiated by isoproterenol 1 or 2 h after the removal of the free lectin. This property was also shared by other insulinomimetic lectins, such as Concanavalin A and wax bean agglutinin. Persistent bioactivation is the consequence of lectin adsorbed to external cell surface determinants in a permanent fashion. This fraction is not internalized, processed, or appreciably dissociated from the cells, since the addition of N-acetyl-D-glucosamine at any time after the onset of wheat germ agglutinin-induced persistent lipogenesis leads to termination. The property of producing persistent bioactivation is not shared by insulin itself, since removal of the unbound hormone results in termination of bioactivation. This study indicates the existence of externally located fat cell surface determinants, which, upon being occupied continuously, produce persistent insulin-like activities. The study also strongly supports the notion that the initial perturbation is sufficient to activate the insulin machinery system, and that internalization and processing of hormone-receptor complexes are the sole pathway for termination."

- https://www.ncbi.nlm.nih.gov/pubmed/6357762 - *PMID: 6357762 DOI: 10.1210/endo-113-6-1921*

Lectins and also stimulate acid production in the stomach resulting in acid reflux. Lectins can bind to mast cells and release histamine. Mast cells are found in the gut and are responsible for destroying and protecting us from pathogenic bacteria. Lectin binding to the mast cell can result in the increase in acid production. The low-carbohydrate diet generally works so well in curing acid reflux because the reduction in consumption of lectin rich foods.

Do dietary lectins cause disease? The evidence is suggestive—and raises interesting possibilities for treatment - David L J Freed,
- https://www.ncbi.nlm.nih.gov/pmc/articles/PMC1115436/

Among the effects observed in the small intestine of lectin fed rodents is stripping away of the mucous coat to expose naked mucosa and overgrowth of the mucosa by abnormal bacteria and protozoa. Lectins also cause discharge of histamine from gastric mast cells, which stimulates acid secretion. So the three main pathogenic factors for peptic ulcer—acid stimulation, failure of the mucous defence layer, and abnormal bacterial proliferation (Helicobacter pylori) are all theoretically linked to lectins. If true, blocking these effects by oligosaccharides would represent an attractive and more physiological treatment for peptic ulcer than suppressing stomach acid. The mucus stripping effect of lectins16 also offers an explanation for the anecdotal finding of many allergists that a "stone age diet," which eliminates most starchy foods and therefore most lectins, protects against common upper respiratory viral infections: without lectins in the throat the nasopharyngeal mucus lining would be more effective as a barrier to viruses.
    - BMJ. 1999 Apr 17; 318(7190): 1023–1024.

Selectins: - combine with immune cells to evoke an inflammatory response. Lectins are also involved and used to adhere the embryo to the uterine wall. (see my book *The Body Map: Reproduction*)

There are ways to reduce the effect of lectins.

- **Cooking** - cooking the food source has a denaturing effect on lectins

- **Fermenting** - some studies find that fermenting the food will reduce the lectin effect by as much as 95%

- **Soaking** - soaking the food source overnight and cooking in fresh water

- **Sprouting** - sprouting beans and grains will substantially reduce the effect of lectins in those sources.

> If you prick us do we not bleed? If you tickle us do we not laugh? If you poison us do we not die? And if you wrong us shall we not revenge?
> — William Shakespeare

"The only time to eat diet food is while you're waiting for the steak to cook." - Julia Child

"A Lie doesn't become truth, wrong doesn't become right and evil doesn't become good, just because it's accepted by a majority."

- Booker T. Washington

Section 3

What are the Intellectual Issues?

In 1911 P&G started advertising their "Crisco" (CRYStalized Cottonseed Oil) as a "healthier alternative to cooking with animal fats. . . and more economical than butter."

X

A Brief History of Medicine and Nutrition

> "The doctor of the future will give no medicine, but will interest his patients in the cause and prevention of disease." -Thomas A. Edison

Edison had the right idea, but drug manufacturers and food companies make this prediction very difficult to fulfill. Change is never, if ever easy and usually takes years for the change to take place. If you look at the history of medicine, you will find that resistance to any change from the accepted norms was hard fought. From blood letting to germs to modern maladies, getting the medical community to accept change has never been easy. Pride, ignorance, arrogance and most of all money, have kept bad practices in place, killing and maiming patients for many decades.

We are living longer than those in earlier ages because we have been able to eradicate or at least control infectious diseases. In the last few years, the recognition that smoking causes various health issues has, to some extent, reduced a number of deaths due to heart disease and cancer.

> ...resistance to path-breaking contributions of obscure scientists is common and "constitutes the single most formidable block to scientific advances." - Nissani, M. (1995). *"The Plight of the Obscure Innovator in Science".*

I look at evidence and outcomes, not someone's credentials and biased opinions. We have been deceived into believing the most absurd things by so-called experts. You will find that studies and statistics can, and have been distorted and manipulated to prove a point of view not in line with the facts and evidence. Food manufacturers and drug companies have a vested interested in promoting ideas that are contrary to sound science.

It is an old saying but still true: "follow the money", you will see that it is the root cause of all the evil, just as Paul told in Timothy:

> *"For the love of money is the root of all evil: which while some coveted after, they have erred from the faith, and pierced themselves through with many sorrows."*- 1 Timothy 6:10.

There are numerous studies, which have been distorted to promote a point of view. The most infamous study which had long-lasting and dire consequences was promoted by Ansel Keys starting in the 1950s. Keys tried to prove his theory that saturated fats cause heart disease. He promoted the idea of low-fat and high carbohydrates as a healthy diet. By manipulating the facts and leaving out information he effectively "proved" his theory to the powers of that day. Keys theory: saturated fats are the cause of heart disease. Since then, the theory has been etched in stone by misleading advertising, misinformed doctors and nutritionists. The drug industry makes BILLIONS of dollars from drugs, which only cover-up and prolong a health issue and do not address the underlying cause of a disease.

Throughout history and even today when an established authority's beliefs are challenged there is an immediate attempt to discredit the person with the dissenting opinion. This vilification is accomplished by the most vile prosecution of the challenger's character. The contradicting proposal itself is avoided because it would mean a thorough investigation of the established authority's own beliefs. Therefore, they must discredit the person by any means possible to maintain the status quo. Change is always met with resistance. The establishment must not be challenged. Only those courageous enough to stand their ground will actually accomplish the change but often the price they pay is enormous; it is the loss of: reputation, career, and finances among other things. This is true in virtually every belief system. In some cases, the belief will not have a deleterious effect on the population at large. However, when it comes to nutrition and the practice of medicine, it can and does affect a very substantial part of the citizenry, especially if the belief is flawed.

For over 50 years, the guidelines for nutrition have been misleading. Obesity, diabetes, and cancer has risen exponentially in the last 50 years because of an established belief that fats and cholesterol are bad and must be avoided, if at all possible. Nevertheless, there is a growing group of doctors, scientists and researchers, who are beginning to question the status quo. These brave men and women are predictably met with extreme prejudice by the medial establishment. I know of three medical doctors who have either been threatened or have lost their license by promoting a diet they know works. Personally, if I followed the advice given by doctors, who have been fed the belief by food and drug companies, I would never have gotten off all the drugs I was taking and would not have regained my health or lost a lot of excess weight and most likely would have died, lost my sight or had a limb cut off as so many unfortunate individuals have done.

Standard of Care

Standard of care is a standard which doctors are held to in caring for their patients by the medical establishment. Going outside of that "acceptable care" scenario could get you fined, jailed or having your license revoked. This is one reason that doctors are fearful of stepping outside of the safe "standard of care" scenario. Throughout history and even today, that standard of care has required doctors to follow the most absurd procedures. A few of these practices in the past included: blood letting, and not washing the hands between patients, practices that today would be seen as barbaric. Unfortunately, it usually takes decades before the establishment changes a practice. The simple practice of washing the hands took 70 years before it became a normal practice by all physicians. In virtually every case, the one who offers an alternative point of view is ridiculed, demonized and run out of the profession.

"Men make history and not the other way around. In periods where there is no leadership, society stands still. Progress occurs when courageous, skillful leaders seize the opportunity to change things for the better. " - Harry S Truman

"Progress is impossible without change, and those who cannot change their minds cannot change anything." - George Bernard Shaw

Bloodletting

For the life of the flesh is in the blood: Leviticus 17:11

Bloodletting was a common practice for almost 3000 years until the late-1800s. Erasistratus in the third century thought that illnesses came from an overabundance of blood. Hippocrates' stated that good health required the balance of the four "humors." The humors were: blood, phlegm, yellow bile and black bile. According to WebMD.com, the practice did sometimes work because it lowered the availability of Heme Iron in the blood after the bloodletting.

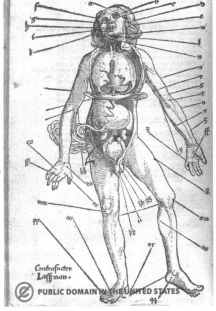

The image on the right shows where to do the bloodletting. The illustration was taken from Field's book of surgery, Strasbourg 1519.

Blood letting is still practiced today by phlebotomists for patients with Hemochromatosis. Hemochromatosis is a genetic disorder where high amounts of Iron are found in the blood. If not corrected the excess iron will get stored in the liver, heart, pancreas and joints causing severe damage and eventually death. It is reported that autopsies have shown people with Alzheimer's, Parkinson, epilepsy, MS and Huntington's had too much iron in the brain. Phlebotomy is done to reduce red blood cells and therefore, excess iron.

177

"Staph thrives on iron compounds, scavenging it from the animals it infects. It obtains most of the iron it needs to grow during infection. Specifically, it prefers a kind of iron found in heme, the molecule in red blood cells that helps carry oxygen. It's as if the bacterium scans its host's menu of iron compounds, hoping to find heme. "Heme iron is the preferred iron source during the initiation of infection," write Skaar and colleagues in the Sept. 10 issue of Science. If no heme is available, the bacterium's chances of thriving may fail."
- https://www.webmd.com/men/news/20040910/bloodlettings-benefits#1

King Charles the II (1630-1685) had about 24 ounces drained from his body before he died. George Washington died after Dr. Brown drained 5 pints of blood from Washington's body. This blood letting was "standard of care" at the time. Would Washington have lived if he had not been bled so profusely anyway? We will never know.

The average adult has about 1.2 to 1.5 gallons approximately 9.5 to 12 pints of blood circulating inside their body.

Bad medical practice has led to other untimely deaths. The author of Little Women, Lousia May Alcott, got sick while attending to the wounded during the Civil War. The doctors at that time gave her large doses of mercury chloride to heal her. The substantial amount of mercury is what most likely lead to her death.

Original Star Trek TV show:

McCoy: What's the matter with you?
Patient: Kidney... Dialysis.
McCoy: Dialysis?! What is this? The Dark Ages? Here! You swallow that and if you have any more problems, just call me!

I believe that someday diabetes may become rare like the practice of bloodletting once the food manufacturers, and the medical profession hear from enough people who have reversed diabetes. In the future we may echo McCoy (Bones) "what is this, the dark ages?" However, if you follow the money, this may be more difficult to achieve. The change will come slowly because there are billions of dollars made each year on diabetic and cholesterol-lowering drugs. The food companies will not be easy to convince that their products contribute to the growing epidemic. For years, doctors have been given erroneous information from drug companies backed up by misleading and fraudulent medical studies. However, if people demand low cost food that is unhealthy, the food manufacturers will provide it. Then who is to be held responsible? We must demand high-quality food. I was in a health-food grocery store, and they were giving free samples of their store brand beef jerky, when I looked at the ingredients, it said low-fat and had massive amounts of sugar and other harmful additions. So much for their health-food reputation! Once you eliminated the prevarication that saturated fat is the problem, then food companies can stop taking the fat out of foods. What happens when you remove the fat? The food becomes flat and boring. How do they overcome this unpleasant tasting food? Add sugar and sometimes MSG. You have now introduced a whole new problem!

Statistics show that the scourge of diabetes is on the rise even among children. At first, I wondered why diabetes was rapidly on the increase. However, I think I now know why there is a sharp increase in diabetes. The issues are: first dietary and second the misunderstanding of how to treat diabetes.

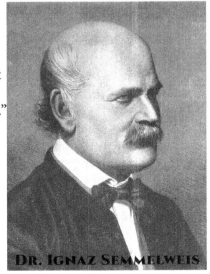

Dr. Semmelweis was an early proponent of washing hands before any procedure. He is described as the "Savior of mothers." He discovered that fatal infections were spread by doctors who did not wash their hands before an examination or procedure. In the mid-1800s, the mortality of puerperal fever also known as "childbed fever" was significantly higher, in fact, three times higher, in the Obstetrical Clinic, than in the midwife's

DR. IGNAZ SEMMELWEIS

179

wards. What he observed was that washing the hands reduced mortality below 1%. Because Semmelweis could not offer an explanation as to why washing hands was so successful, the medical community rejected his advice. Some doctors even mocked Dr. Semmelweis for suggesting it. Dr. Semmelweis died long before Louis Pasteur discovered the existence of germs. His prognosis was correct, only he did not know why. An example of ignorance and pride that kept the medical community from recognizing a medical fact that could have saved countless lives. Dr. Semmelweis was in conflict most of the time with the "accepted" opinion of his time also known as "belief perseverance". Getting the community to change their beliefs proved almost impossible. It was during this time that they held to a barbaric procedure known as blood letting. This was based on ignorance, which held to the theory of dyscrasia, a Greek term for bad mixture. It was believed that the imbalance in the blood was the cause of most maladies.

Semmelweis was eventually sent to an asylum where the attendants beat him. I don't know why they beat him, but he got an infection from the beating and soon died from the infection. It is interesting to note that James Garfield did not die from the assassin's bullet he died from an infection. The infection was the result of the doctors who were not in the practice of washing their hands in 1881 when Garfield was shot.

Louis Pasteur (1822-1895) Pasteur was also persecuted by the medical community for his ideas on germ theory. He was eventually proven correct. The medical profession had no clue that there were such things as microorganisms. In the 1880s, Pasteur showed that heating wine would inactivate harmful microorganisms that caused the wine to sour. This heating process, pasteurization, is named after Louis Pasteur. The process of heating a liquid just below the boiling point is a common practice today. Pasteurization of milk became law in the early 20th century. Louis Pasteur is not at fault for pasteurizing milk; it was a result of the poor sanitation of dairies at the time. The process of pasteurization not only kills any good bacteria, it destroys much of the nutritional value as well. The following is a quote about the dangers of pasteurizing and homogenization of milk.

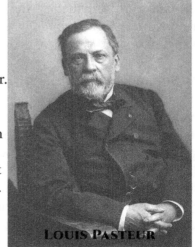

LOUIS PASTEUR

"Pasteurization destroys enzymes, diminishes vitamin content, denatures fragile milk proteins, destroys vitamins C, B12 and B6, kills beneficial bacteria, promotes pathogens and is associated with allergies, increased tooth decay, colic in infants, growth problems in children,osteoporosis, arthritis, heart disease and cancer.

Homogenization makes fat molecules in milk smaller and they become "capsules" for substances that are able to bypass digestion. Proteins that would normally be digested in the stomach are not broken down and instead they are absorbed into the bloodstream."

- by PreventDisease.com © 1999-2018. All Rights Reserved.

Heart Disease was largely unknown until the late 1800s. According to Center for Disease Control (CDC) it wasn't until the 1920s that heart attacks became the leading cause of death in the United States. This can be traced to a change in the diet with the introduction of Vegetable oils, incorrectly named because these oils come from seeds like cotton, corn and other seeds. People in the early 20th century were told that Crisco® Oil was healthier than butter, lard or tallow. Crisco® was introduced in 1911. Just a few short years later, heart attacks became the leading cause of death. Was this coincidence?

Wilhelm Normann (1870 - 1939)

Normann discovered he could hydrogenate liquid oils in 1901, this later became known as trans fats when applied to vegetable oils. His work influenced the production of margarine and vegetable shortening. Proctor & Gamble acquired the US rights to the Normann's patent. They then started producing PHOs (partially hydrogenated oil). William Proctor and his brother in-law used cotton seed oil in the making of soap and candles. Since the meat-packing industry controlled the price of lard and tallow, the two decided to use cotton seed oil. They discovered that by hydrogenating the oil it would become solid and had the appearance of lard. Since the candle business was diminishing they decided to sell the new product as a food. In 1911, P&G started advertising their "Crisco" (CRYStalized Cottonseed Oil) as a "healthier alternative to cooking with animal fats. . . and more economical than butter."

This contrivance, along with other vegetable oils are bad for many reasons. The chemical reaction in the body to this brew will affect the body in detrimental ways. A simple explanation is how it affects the production of prostacyclin.

"Prostacyclin is a prostaglandin member of the eicosanoid family of lipid molecules. It inhibits platelet activation and is also an effective vasodilator." - Wikipedia

In simple language, prostacyclin is a signaling molecule that keeps platelets from forming in the blood and is synthesized in the endothelial cells (cells lining the veins and arteries) it also dilates the blood vessels. Without prostacyclin clotting begins to form.

Elliot P. Joslin, MD (1869-1962)

Joslin is known as the father of diabetic treatment. Joslin wrote *Diabetic Manual — for the Doctor and Patient*. You can read his book (187 pages) (at the time I am writing this book at) **https://archive.org/details/diabeticmanualfo00joslrich/**

He had a list of 29 foods that were strictly forbidden. Among those foods were: sugars, farinaceous foods and starches (whatever ever will produce a flour or ground meal), bread, pasta, all sweet and dried fruits, all sweet wines and many more. He is the founder of the Joslin Diabetes Center still in operation today.

> "Despite being controversial recommendations based on weak scientific evidence, the United States Department of Agriculture (USDA) created in 1980 a food pyramid and placed carbohydrates at its base. This national nutritional experiment contributed, as we know now, to the increased prevalence of obesity."
>
> – Osama Hamdy, Medical Director, Joslin Diabetes Center, Harvard Medical School, Nutrition Revolution: *The End of the High Carbohydrates Era for Diabetes Prevention and Management*

Sir William Osler (1849 - 1919)
Wrote one of the most famous medical books of all time *Principles and Practices of Medicine,* published in 1892. He included in that book the Banting Diet a low-carb high fat diet (LCHF).

"The greater the ignorance the greater the dogmatism."
Dr. William Osler

"One of the first duties of the physician is to educate the masses not to take medicine". Dr. William Osler

"The good physician treats the disease; the great physician treats the patient who has the disease." Dr. William Osler

Read more at:
https://www.brainyquote.com/authors/william_osler

William Banting - (1796-1878)

Banting was in his mid-60s, 5' 6" tall and obese over 200 lbs. In 1863 after he lost weight, he wrote a pamphlet titled Letter on Corpulence. The pamphlet was a personal testimony of his success at losing weight (52 lbs.).

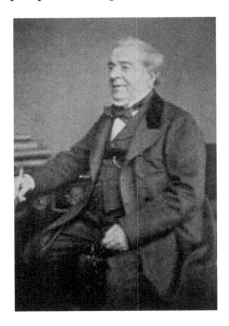

Banting had very strict rules: no bread, sugar, beer and potatoes. He ate meat, vegetables and fish. Dr. William Harvey was the doctor who prescribed the diet to Banting. Today, Dr. Tim Noakes (From South Africa) calls his keto style diet "the Banting Diet"

"My diminished girth, in tailor phraseology, was hardly conceivable even by my own friends, or my respected medical adviser, until I put on my former clothing, over what I now wear, which is a thoroughly convincing proof of the remarkable change."

"The point to keep in mind is that you don't lose fat because you cut calories; you lose fat because you cut out the foods that make you fat-the carbohydrates." — Gary Taubes "more luxurious and liberal, independent of its blessed effect, but when it is proved to be more healthful, the comparisons are simply ridiculous."

"I am very much better both bodily and mentally and pleased to believe that I hold the reins of health and comfort in my own hands."

"It is simply miraculous and I am thankful to Almighty Providence for directing me through an extraordinary chance to the care of a man who worked such a change in so short a time."

"For the sake of argument and illustration I will presume that certain articles of ordinary diet, however beneficial in youth, are prejudicial in advanced life, like beans to a horse, whose common ordinary food is hay and corn. It may be useful food occasionally, under peculiar circumstances, but detrimental as a constancy. I will, therefore, adopt the analogy, and call such food human beans. The items from which I was advised to abstain as much as possible were: Bread . . butter...sugar, beer, and potatoes, which had been the main (and, I thought, innocent) elements of my existence, or at all events they had for many years been adopted freely. These, said my excellent adviser, contain starch and saccharine matter, tending to create fat, and should be avoided altogether." - quotes by William Banting

Canadian explorer Vilhjalmur Stefansson (1879–1962)

Stefansson lived with the Inuit Eskimos in Alaska. He found that the Inuit diet was over 90% meat and fish. Yet, the Inuit were quite healthy.

"For I had published in 1913, on pages 140-142 of My Life with the Eskimo, an account of how some natives and I became ill when we had to go two or three weeks on lean meat, caribou so skinny that there was no appreciable fat behind the eyes or in the marrow. So when Dr. DuBois suggest that I start the meat period by eating as many large quantities as I possibly could of chopped fatless muscle, I predicted trouble." - *Adventures in Diet Part 2* - Vilhjalmur Stefansson - Harper's Monthly Magazine, December 1935.

Health of the Inuit as observed by Stefansson:
The Inuit had perfect dental health, no signs of osteoporosis, no cancer, no heart disease, cardiovascular disease, no type 2 diabetes and no obesity.

Why are we still talking about saturated fats being the root cause of the many diseases? Could it be avarice on the part of the food and drug companies?

> "Pasteurized milk has up to a 66 percent loss of vitamins A, D and E. Vitamin C loss usually exceeds 50 percent. Heat affects water soluble vitamins and can make them 38 percent to 80 percent less effective. Vitamins B6 and B12 are completely destroyed during pasteurization. Pasteurization also destroys beneficial enzymes, antibodies and hormones. Pasteurization destroys lipase (an enzyme that breaks down fat), which impairs fat metabolism and the ability to properly absorb fat soluble vitamins A and D. (The dairy industry is aware of the diminished vitamin D content in commercial milk, so they fortify it with a form of this vitamin.)"
>
> "Milk straight from the cow contains cream, which rises to the top. Homogenization is a process that breaks up the fat globules and evenly distributes them throughout the milk so that they do not rise. This process unnaturally increases the surface area of fat exposing it to air, in which oxidation occurs and increases the susceptibility to spoilage. Homogenization has been linked to heart disease and atherosclerosis."
>
> - *Milk: It Does a Body Good?* July 7, 2003 By Lori Lipinski - from *Wise Traditions in Food, Farming and the Healing Arts*, the quarterly magazine of the Weston A. Price Foundation, Spring 2003.

Weston A. Price (1870 - 1948) - DDS

Weston A Price was a dentist. His book *Nutrition and Physical Degeneration* is his unique study of the importance of whole food nutrition, and the ill effects caused by processed foods. Dr. Price traveled across the world visiting isolated primitive people (those who have not adopted the modern diet) What he found is astounding: no tooth decay, healthy bodies and minds free from disease and illnesses common to us today. Today his mission continues with the Weston Price Foundation. According to the Weston Foundation, the diets of these isolated people did not contain: refined sugar, white flour, pasteurized, homogenized skim milk, vegetable oils or other toxic additives.

Find the Weston Price Foundation at: https://www.westonaprice.org/

In 1945, Dr. Weston Price described "a new vitamin-like activator" that played an influential role in the utilization of minerals, protection from tooth decay, growth and development, reproduction, protection against heart disease and the function of the brain. Using a chemical test, he determined that this compound—which he called Activator X—occurred in the butterfat, organs and fat of animals consuming rapidly growing green grass, and also in certain sea foods such as fish eggs.

Read the whole article at:
https://www.westonaprice.org/health-topics/abcs-of-nutrition/on-the-trail-of-the-elusive-x-factor-a-sixty-two-year-old-mystery-finally-solved/

Dr. Christiaan Eijkman (1858-1930)

Dutch physician Christiaan Eijkman, was sent to Java to discover why people were dying from a disease named beriberi. Symptoms of beriberi include: muscular atrophy, paralysis and death. Initially, it was thought the disease came from a virus or bacteria. This theory was based on Louis Pasteur's work on germs.

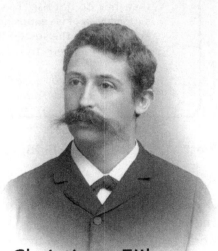

Christiaan Eijkman

Eijkman's experiments involved feeding chickens white polished rice. The chickens came down with beriberi and died. Because white rice was more expensive, he switched to unprocessed rice. When he switched to unpolished rice, the chickens thrived. He initially called the ingredient "the anti-beriberi factor." Eventually, it was determined that the skin of unpolished rice had something that was removed when converted to polished white rice. He called the discovery "vital amine." A chemist, Casimir Funk, shortened and coined the term vitamin. The vitamin in this case was later named vitamin B1 (thiamine).

It is my contention that today food companies are practicing the same ill-advised conduct. Removing from food "God given" nutrients and replacing it with sugar and man-made concoctions! It is no wonder we have the rampant disease crisis that we have today. However, we never seem to learn that God gave man everything he needed to survive and thrive. Are the food and drug industries systematically destroying our health all in the name of profit and greed? We are ignoring the common sense of those who came before us like Dr. Eijkman! There are many factors involved in the destruction of health: poor farming practices, consuming excess sugar and carbohydrates, chemicals in the environment, pasteurization, just to name a few.

Dr. George V. Mann (1917-2013)- MD, and professor of biochemistry

In his book *Coronary Heart Disease: The Dietary Sense and Nonsense* he exposes the fraudulent claims and commercial exploitation by the manufacturers of margarine, and vegetable oils and how the regulatory agencies "turned a blind eye." He also had a contrary view about heart disease, consumption of foods like eggs; meats are not the direct cause of CHD (coronary heart disease). Dr. Mann lost a $60,000 funding in 1968 by the NIH (National Institutes of Health) because of his beliefs on cholesterol.

In the 1960s, Dr. Mann visited the Masai tribe in Kenya, Africa. He found that their diet consisted of over 60% saturated fat. Dr. Mann did examinations on over 1500 Masai. He found no diabetes, no heart disease and no cancer.

Ancel Keys, PhD - A name that will live in infamy.

In the 1960s there was a rapidly increasing number of cases of heart disease. Something had to be done immediately the fear of a heart attack was at a peak, and then came Ancel Keys.

Keys' original claim to fame was for the formulation of the k-ration used in the military. He had a BA in economics and a PhD in fish physiology. He was not a medical doctor and did not take nutritional courses in college. However, Keys is most infamous for his "Seven Countries Study" this study assumed to show that serum cholesterol was ultimately responsible for coronary heart disease. Nevertheless, he did not include all of his findings from the complete study of 22 countries. The countries which did not fit his hypothesis were left out. The truth was that there was no correlation. Since 1900, coronary heart disease increased dramatically. This was very alarming to the population; something had to be done. In 1952, Keys presented his diet-heart hypothesis in which he linked fat consumption to heart disease. In 1956, Keys went on television and proclaimed that in order to prevent heart disease everyone should adopt a low-fat diet. He suggested cutting down on eggs, butter, lard and beef. Consequently, the American government followed his advice. We have been held hostage to that belief ever since. The question that must be asked is: if people have been eating saturated fat for centuries without consequence, why would it cause heart disease now? We can clearly see an inverse relationship between the consumption of saturated fat, which has decreased and at the same time period heart disease, obesity, diabetes and many more debilitating diseases are increasing. Keys will go down in history as the villain who fraudulently convinced the world that saturated fat and cholesterol were the reason for many fatal diseases.

"Contrary to common beliefs, the current recommendations to reduce saturated fats have no scientific basis. I'm not the only one saying this. You must have heard of the book called 'The Big Fat Surprise' by Nina Teicholz. She shook up the nutrition world, but she got it right."

"Did you know that the seven countries studies that actually had a straight line between fat intake and CVD is fudged. I'm using the word fudged because 23 countries participated in that study and they took the seven best that fitted that line, and that's what's there. If you go through the literature, you will find that they chose the seven that fitted the line. The nutrition field has been distorted."

— DR. Salim Yusuf
the Marion W. Burke Chair in Cardiovascular Disease at McMaster University Medical School. He is a cardiologist and epidemiologist In 2014, he was awarded the Canada Gairdner Wightman Award and was inducted into the Canadian Medical Hall of Fame.[

The 1977 US Dietary Goals for Americans (USDGA)

> "What right has the federal government to propose that the American people conduct a vast nutritional experiment, with themselves as subjects, on the strength of so little evidence that it will do them any good?"
>
> Phillip Handles, President of the National Academy of Sciences, Congressional testimony in response to Dietary Goals for the United States, 1980

This nefarious guideline promoted the idea of a diet high in carbohydrates – requiring six to 11 servings a day of cereals and grains and up to 5 daily servings of fruits and vegetables – and very low in fat, especially saturated fat. Since that time, there has been NO study or research to prove that the diet actually reduces obesity or heart disease the opposite is a fact. Since that time, obesity, heart disease, diabetes and other illnesses have increased exponentially! Yet, there is a refusal in the face of overwhelming evidence to the contrary, that the guideline should be reversed. I will attempt to show in layman's terms exactly how the body reacts and processes the food we eat. The term lipophobia was coined to describe the fear of fats.

> "The evidence – both from experiments and from field surveys – indicates that cholesterol content, per se, of all natural diets has no significant effect on either the cholesterol level or the development of atherosclerosis in man." - *Symposium on Atherosclerosis*
> - The National Academy Press

Dr. Richard Mackarness

Dr. Mackarness wrote a book called *Eat Fat and Grow Slim* in 1958. It is amazing that the LC/HF diet has been around for a long time. Yet, we were not made aware of it, why?

> "A story about the Jack Spratts of medicine [was] told recently by Dr. Charles H. Best, co-discoverer of insulin. He had been invited to a conference of heart specialists in North America. On the eve of the meeting, out of respect for the fat-clogs-the-arteries theory,

the delegates sat down to a special banquet served without fats. It was unpalatable but they all ate it as a duty. Next morning Best looked round the breakfast room and saw these same specialists— all in the 40-60 year old, coronary age group—happily tucking into eggs, bacon, buttered toast and coffee with cream."
— Richard Mackarness, Eat Fat And Grow Slim

"If a fat man stops eating carbohydrate, he makes little pyruvic acid and removes the stimulus to his "fat organ" to make fat. By eating fat and protein he by-passes his metabolic block. To put it another way: obesity may be regarded as a compensatory overgrowth of the fatty tissues providing for an increased use of fat by a body incapable of using carbohydrate properly. Feed a fat man fat and protein in place of starch and sugar and he will deal with that quite well, drawing on his stores of body fat in the process. Paradoxically, he will eat fat and grow thinner. He will also feel well because he will no longer be subjecting his body to starvation and he will be tackling the fundamental cause of his obesity which is not over-eating but a defect in the complex biochemical machinery of his body."

Journal of Biological Chemistry, in 1955, as follows:
"Fasting or feeding a high-fat diet abolished lipogenesis (fat formation) in adipose tissue and reduced glucose oxidation markedly lipogenesis increased to the highest levels on a high-carbohydrate, fat-free diet."

- Dr. Richard Mackarness - *Eat Fat and Grow Slim*

John Yudkin

Yudkin studied biochemistry and physiology, before taking up medicine. He wrote a book in 1972 *Pure, White and Deadly* about the dangers of sugar in the diet. Ancel Keys attacked Yudkin for his beliefs calling it "a mountain of nonsense." Keys and the sugar industry were successful in the destruction of Yudkin's reputation. You see, Keys had been funded by the sugar industry since the 1940s. Now, Yudkin's belief has been proven to be correct. I highly recommend that you get a copy of his book. It is available as an e-book on Amazon. Robert Lustig has taken up the cause and reissued the book with a forward written by himself. Dr. Lustig has written his own book called *Fat Chance: Beating the Odds Against Sugar, Processed Food, Obesity, and Disease.* I highly recommend his book as well. You can find many YouTube videos by Dr. Lustig, which present mountains of information and statistics on the subject.

Dr. Cristin Kearns, DDS

Kearns is a dentist who became a researcher after attending a conference on oral health where conference speakers touted the type of diet recommended for diabetic patients. The handouts told the dentists that diabetic patients could lose weight and eat fewer saturated fats but nothing about sugar consumption. As a dentist she saw first-hand the result of sugar consumption: tooth decay. She began research into the reasons why sugar was not mentioned. What she found was disturbing. She had to find the answers, after several months she discovered the archives of a bankrupt sugar company. The documents showed that sugar industry was actively involved in a campaign to deceive the public about the dangers of sugar consumption by redirecting the attention of the public to evils of saturated fats. This deed was accomplished by two Harvard nutritionists, Dr. Fredrick Stare and Mark Hegsted both worked closely with the Sugar Research Foundation. In 1967, they published their beliefs in the New England Journal of Medicine, which stated that Americans should eat a low-fat diet.

Does anyone believe that sugar filled cereals are good for you? Or sugar filled sodas with an overabundance of sodium will not generate fat in the body? Listening to the ads you would think you must get your required daily vitamins from this high-carbohydrate sugar infused morsels. I have a DVD of old cigarette commercials, which speak of the smooth flavor, how much you will enjoy smoking their brand you would think that you could not live without smoking. They even had the audacity to use the children's cartoon characters Fred Flintstones and Barney Rubble to promote their product. The cigarette companies even whet as far as adding sugar to their product to make it more enjoyable. The problem is that smoking causes whole plethora diseases and adverse chemical reactions in the body. However, you would never know that from their commercials. Today sugar laced foods pick up where smoking left off. Doctors are starting to wake up and speak out against low-fat/high-carbohydrate diets.

However, remember each one of us is unique, some, including George Burns did not get cancer from his cigar smoking. Therefore, we cannot conclude that cigarette smoking will positively give you cancer, there are many who smoked all their life without getting cancer. The path to good health is not always obvious. It is obvious that something about George Burns kept him from getting the dreaded cancer.

Dr. Fredrick Stare M.D. (1910-2002)

Dr. Stare from Harvard University was against the health food and organic food movements. Dr. Stare received massive funding by Coca-Cola, National Soft drinks Association among others. He was paid by the sugar industry (in the form of grants) to protect its products and their profits.

> 51 years ago, a bribe and a lie involving Harvard scientists Drs. Frederick Stare and Mark Hegsted led to one of the worst scandals ever in human nutrition… and you're still paying for it with your health to this day.- A. O'Connor. *Sugar Backers Paid to Shift Blame to Fat*. The New York Times. September 13, 2016: A1

Professor Tim Noakes MD

To show how arrogant and resistant to change people can be, the professor was dragged into court by a dietitian with the Association for Dietetics in South Africa for sending a tweet suggesting a low-carb diet for young children. Like the advice the dietitians have been giving is working so well!

I realized that carbohydrates gave me diabetes, I was addicted to bread and sports drinks.
– Timothy Noakes

There is a growing number of doctors, researchers and dietitians which are rebelling against the guidelines and coming out in favor of evidenced-based health care.

Dr. Vinayak Prasad, MD.

Dr. Prasad and his team reviewed 10 years of articles published in the prestigious New England Journal of Medicine. The intent of the review was to identify medical practices that don't work. Their book *Ending Medical Reversal: Improving Outcomes, Saving Lives* -Johns Hopkins University Press. Both Dr. Prasad and Dr. Adam Cifu have the conclusions from their findings. The premise of the book is to do a better job of recommending practices that actually work.

Quotes from an article:
Researchers Identify 146 Contemporary Medical Practices Offering No Net Benefits
Articles appear in Mayo Clinic Proceedings, Volume 88, Issue 8 (August 2013), published by Elsevier.

"While the next breakthrough is surely worth pursuing, knowing whether what we are currently doing is right or wrong is equally crucial for sound patient care." - Dr. Prasad

"A large proportion of current medical practice, 40%, was found to offer no benefits in our survey of 10 years of the New England Journal of Medicine. These 146 practices are medical reversals. They weren't just practices that once worked, and have now been improved upon; rather, they never worked. They were instituted in error, never helped patients, and have eroded trust in medicine." - Dr. Prasad

"Health care costs now threaten the entire economy. Our investigation suggests that much of what we are doing today simply doesn't help patients. Eliminating medical reversal may help address the most pressing problem in health care today. - Dr. Prasad

In my opinion, the term "practicing medicine" is fundamentally just that, practicing. Since the human body is so extremely complex, each one of us is different, and our environment is constantly changing it would be impossible for any man or woman to diagnose and treat illnesses with a perfect record every time, there too many variables. However, it is insane to continue to prescribe a treatment which is, for all practical purposes, ineffective on one side and often deadly on the other. In this book I hope to provoke you to research, to question and to learn what is working and what is not. Many times the standard of practice is "dead" wrong and must be corrected. Dr. Prasad is absolutely correct; some of the practices are ineffective and are costing billions of dollars and a massive loss of limbs, quality of life and life itself.

Rather than take the easy road and follow the directives of the medical establishment, some courageous doctors are taking a second look at the facts and are following an evidence-based practice. For me, rather than take advice at face value, I would like to see proof for the recommended care.

Health Epidemics

The Black Plague (Bubonic plague) - 45 million+ deaths

In the 1300s, the plague was introduced into Europe by ships entering the Sicilian port of Messina. The disease was so infectious that it easily spread through the air as well as from infected fleas and rats. They did not have the knowledge we have today and the plague was not abated until they required sailors to stay on the ship for up to 40 days or for a "quarantino" the beginning of the use of the word quarantine.

Smallpox - 3 out of 10 who contracted the disease died.

An interesting story from history about adaptive immunity comes from our first President, George Washington. When George was 19 years old, he went to Barbados with his brother Lawrence. Lawrence had tuberculosis, and it was suggested that they go to Barbados. Upon arriving in Barbados, they were invited to the home of Gedney Clarke, a family friend and wealthy merchant. George was reluctant to attend because there was smallpox in their home. His fears were realized when he contracted the disease. He was able to overcome smallpox and became well again. (This is the reason he had noticeable scars on his face.)

During the Revolutionary War, there was an outbreak of smallpox. This gave the British the upper hand because they had already survived an outbreak in England and were already immune to the disease. It is speculated that the British were involved in a type of chemical warfare, by attempting to spread the disease. Washington had a dilemma, if he inoculated the men they would be out for some period giving the British the upper hand, if he did not he would lose more men to the malady. Washington's decision to inoculate the men proved to be the right decision. He could now fight with a full complement of men.

According to medical history smallpox was responsible for more deaths than any other infectious disease. Smallpox was totally eradicated worldwide by 1980; however, the virus still exists under lock and key in Atlanta, Georgia and Russia. That is a very scary, since it could be released now and many of the younger generations would be susceptible to the disease.

Spanish Flu (1918) - 40+ million deaths

Influenza (flu) attacks the respiratory system. The flu outbreaks happen every year and according to Centers for Disease Control, and Prevention (CDC) says that it results in between 3,000 to 49,000 deaths each year. Those most vulnerable among us are those over 65 years old, and some have medical conditions like asthma, diabetes, heart disease and other maladies. It is told that more soldiers died from the flu than were killed in the war. Some people acquired immunity to the virus.

During the time I am researching and writing this book there is a new respiratory "flu" called the Wuhan flu or covid-19. It's effects are nowhere near the Spanish flu but the panic is nonetheless more devastating. We are told that many deaths that were directly attributable to C-19 were cause by other things and contracted by mostly those who have other illnesses. Over 92% who contract the disease recover, some don't even know they had it. At this point the panic has caused by far more economic destruction than deaths of healthy people. Some took the opportunity to impose harsh, unreasonable rules. Only time will tell what the real effect of this disease will be.

Aids - 25 million+ deaths

We did not know about AIDS just a few decades ago. It was first identified in 1981. Autoimmune diseases, used to fight viruses and other invaders, let the immune system, attack the body. AIDS actually shuts down the immune system.

"HIV (human immunodeficiency virus) is a virus that attacks cells that help the body fight infection, making a person more vulnerable to other infections and diseases. It is spread by contact with certain bodily fluids of a person with HIV, most commonly during unprotected sex (sex without a condom or HIV medicine to prevent or treat HIV), or through sharing injection drug equipment. If left untreated, HIV can lead to the disease AIDS (acquired immunodeficiency syndrome)." - https://www.HIV.gov

Obesity and heart disease - 100 million+ deaths

We have an health epidemic today which I believe can be corrected. The cost from all the outcomes of obesity is astronomical and climbing. Speaking of cholesterol and heart disease read what renown heart specialist Michael DeBakey said:

> **"If you say cholesterol is the cause, how do you explain the other 60 percent to 70 percent with heart disease who don't have a high cholesterol?"**
>
> - Michael De Bakey,
>   JAMA, 189:655-659, (1964)

Obesity has taken more lives than all previous epidemics. Unlike epidemics that kill in days (Black Death), weeks (influenza), or years (AIDS), obesity kills over decades - *The Fat Switch* - Richard Johnson M.D.

> *Reminder: I am researching the issues; I am not a licensed doctor and do not practice medicine. You need to contact a practitioner who has the right to diagnose and treat your issue, see appendix B for a list of practitioners. Nothing in this book should be taken as medical advice.*

My hypothesis

It has been my opinion (conspiracy theory if you prefer) that organizations that say they want to cure diseases like Cancer, Diabetes and Heart disease, in reality, do not want a cure for their named disease. The cure would mean that the enormous amounts of money they get through their fund-raising campaigns and donations from industry would be cut off, and it would be the end of their existence. This would be good for those with the disease but not for those organizations getting the funding. The fact that we know in most cases that diabetes can be reversed, we should see a change in Diabetes Foundation's recommendations. ...I am not holding my breath. I will give further evidence in the next chapter on Health and Politics.

> **"The thing that bugs me is that the people think the FDA is protecting them - it isn't. What the FDA is doing and what the public thinks it's doing are as different as night and day."** -Herbert L. Ley, Jr. 10th Commissioner and head of the U.S. Food and Drug Administration (FDA).

We are now in a crisis of Biblical proportions. We cannot sustain the massive debt load that these diseases put on the American people, let alone the pain and suffering physically, financially and mentally of those with the disease and their families. I believe there is an answer, but the powers that be must look at the results of their recommendations realistically and see that they have not worked since they were adopted decades ago. We must insist that changes be made before another generation is subjected to injurious advice brought to us by bad science and biased research. I know of many instances, including my own, where diabetes can be overcome and the drugs are no longer necessary when following an appropriate diet. When are we going to wake up? We can prove that smoking is one of the causes of heart diseases because of the chemical reactions in the body. The reduction in heart-related deaths we have seen in the last years has, at least in part, to do with the reduction in smoking. Will we see a further reduction in deaths by heart and diabetes diseases when we follow a better diet? Only time will tell. The good news is, there are doctors and researchers that are waking up to the truth of the matter, some at great cost for going against the establishment. There may be hope for us yet.

"In fact, two slices of whole wheat bread increase blood sugar to a higher level than a candy bar does. And then, after about two hours, your blood sugar plunges and you get shaky, your brain feels foggy, you're hungry."
— William Davis -author of *Wheat Belly*

"Researchers have known for some time now that the cornerstone of all degenerative conditions, including brain disorders, is inflammation. But what they didn't have documented until now are the instigators of that inflammation—the first missteps that prompt this deadly reaction. And what they are finding is that gluten, and a high-carbohydrate diet for that matter, are among the most prominent simulators of inflammatory pathways that reach the brain." — David Perlmutter - author of *Grain Brain*

"It's more important to understand the imbalances in your body's basic systems and restore balance, rather than name the disease and match the pill to the ill."
— Mark Hyman, M.D. author of *Food Fix: How to Save Our Health, Our Economy, Our Communities, and Our Planet--One Bite at a Time*

"The great enemy of truth is very often not the lie--deliberate, contrived and dishonest--but the myth--persistent, persuasive and unrealistic. Too often we hold fast to the cliches of our forebears. We subject all facts to a prefabricated set of interpretations. We enjoy the comfort of opinion without the discomfort of thought - John F. Kennedy

- from the *Commencement Address at Yale University*, June 11 1962

XI

Politics and Our Health

"It's easier to fool people than to convince them that they have been fooled."
- Mark Twain (unverified)

"Seventy percent of the federal budget is for Medicare, Medicaid, and Social Security. By 2042, 100% of the federal budget will be required to pay for Medicare and Medicaid, leaving nothing for defense, transportation, education, agriculture, environment, or any of the government's other basic services.

...The Diabetes Prevention Program showed that a structured lifestyle-change program could reduce the progression to diabetes by 58%, working better than any other known treatment."

Mark Hayman, MD

If you analyze history, you will find that the prognosticators of doom are **virtually always wrong**. Al Gore in his speech, dubbed, "*Earth Has A Fever*," predicted, in 2006 that the North Pole would be "ice-free" by around 2013 because of alleged "man-made global warming. I could go on quoting many doomsday predictions, which at no time materialized. There are many predictions, which end up costing us billions of dollars and never accomplished a thing. Politics and religion also cause massive destruction; wars, famine and death. For example, look at death by famine just in the 20th century. (from https://listverse.com/2013/04/10/10-terrible-famines-in-history/By Andrew Fitzgerald April 10, 2013.):

Russian Famine of 1921 - **5 Million dead**.
> *Man-Made Famine*
> Because of the multiple civil wars and the violent revolution in 1917 it was a difficult time for the Russian people. Bolshevik soldiers often forced peasants to give them their food. Because of that many peasants stopped growing crops they would not eat. The peasants began eating the seed since they would not eat what they had grown. [a good case against socialism]

Soviet Famine of 1932 - **10 Million dead**
> *Man-Made famine*
> Josef Stalin forcibly took the land from peasants and turned them into collectives. When the peasants hid their crops, Stalin sent out search parties and destroyed the hidden crops including seed that would be used for the next year.

Bengal Famine of 1943 - **7 million dead**
both Man-Made and Natural causes:
A majority of food was imported from Burma, but with the
Japanese take over the trading stopped. Also weather destroyed
90% of their crops because of rain and fungus. And because there
was an influx of Burmese fleeing Burma there simply was not
enough food.

Vietnamese Famine of 1945 - **2 Million dead**
Man-Made Famine & Natural causes
The Japanese were expansing into Indochina and
Vietnam. Then the French sided with the Japanese. This resulted
in a shift from farming to war-materials also there was a drought
and flooding which caused the famine.

Great Chinese Famine 1958 - **43 million dead**.
Man-Made famine
This was due to the "Great leap forward" which outlawed owning
of Private land. Millions of agricultural workers were forced to
work in factories.

North Korean Famine 1994-98 - **3 Million Dead**.
Man-Made Famine
Kim Jung Il implemented "military first" needs of the military
came before the people. His unwillingness to import food and
torrential rains in 1995 caused mass malnutrition and starvation.

Now because of fraudulent information, the government has
recommended a diet which has proven to be a disaster. We have shown
that disease, and obesity is on an exponential rise as a result of their
suggested diet plan.

If you think that the politicians, the drug, and food companies have your
best health interests in mind, I have a rude awaking for you, they do
not! Politicians need money to get re-elected; food and drug companies
need customers for their products, and universities need money for their
existence. Do you begin to see the potential for bad policies and biased
research? Drug companies are very willing to give massive amounts of

money to politicians and universities who will follow their advice. Doctors are given virtually NO training on nutrition (I have heard medical doctors say they had less than one day of nutritional training in medical school). How can a doctor give advice on nutrition? What they are taught in medical school is how to address an illness with drugs NOT how to reverse a disease. It is my experience that doctors do not concern themselves with why a patient has a particular disease, only "how can I relieve the symptoms" or "how can I slow down the progress of the illness".

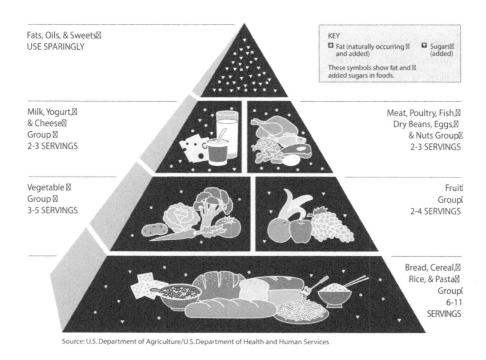

Food Guide Pyramid
A Guide to Daily Food Choices

Source: U.S. Department of Agriculture/U.S. Department of Health and Human Services

Do you think studies that come out of universities or researchers that get large amounts of funding from food and drug companies will be unbiased? The obvious answer is a resounding, **NO!**

> For every complex problem there is an answer that is clear, simple, and wrong. - H. L. Mencken

Nina Teicholz in her book *The Big Fat Surprise: Why Butter, Meat and Cheese Belong in a Healthy Diet* points out foods that we have been told are bad for us are the very foods that can reverse obesity, diabetes and heart disease. I can personally attest to that fact. There is a growing number of people who are experiencing the benefits of returning to a diet our forefathers ate before all the misinformation about cholesterol and saturated fats. Teicholz goes on to say that in the early 1900s, there were only a few who died of heart disease but by the 1950s, heart disease became the number-one killer. In her book, she sites that in 1961 when The American Heart Association (AHA from now on) recommended a low fat, low cholesterol diet only one in seven Americans were obese. By 2001 that number had leaped to one in three were obese. During the same time, diabetes had risen from less than one percent to over eleven percent, and heart disease is still the leading cause of death. However, the number of deaths from heart disease has declined in recent years; I believe because so many have quit smoking.

The American Heart Association got its real start in 1948 when they were given $1.5 million by Proctor and Gamble as a result of a promotion on the radio show *Truth or Consequences.*

> The AHA remained small until the 1940s when it was selected for support by Proctor & Gamble, via their PR firm, from a list of applicant charities. Proctor & Gamble gave $1.5 million from its radio show, Truth or Consequences, allowing the organization to go national.
>
> Tye, Larry (1998). The Father of Spin: Edward L. Bernays & the Birth of Public Relations. p. 74.

Not surprising that the AHA said that Crisco (Crystallized Cottonseed Oil, made by Proctor & Gamble) is healthier than butter. We now know that trans-fat from vegetable oils is very unhealthy even deadly!

"Follow the money".

Ancel Keys, a name that will live in infamy, and will become known as the most villainous health researchers in American history. Keys had a biased and deceptive practice of leaving out a major parts of his research to prove his very flawed hypothesis. He attempted to show that dietary saturated fat causes cardiovascular heart disease and should be avoided. Over the years, anyone who dare contradict this premise has been silenced, being cut off from grants, and having their influence disappear.

> "So what is the answer to increased health and vigor? Eating more or fewer foods is not the answer. The key lies in knowing what to eat. You need to know how to obtain the essential micro and macro nutrients and the amount needed daily. This is a very important point that the food pyramid system fails to consider. The reason for this is that current nutritional thinking pushes a philosophy of food groups and not the essential micro and macro-nutrients you need. When you are eating to get sufficient nutrients, you will not ask how many food servings to eat but the amount of the actual micro and macro-nutrients needed."
>
> Luan Pho. *Health and Vitality Truths* . Luan Q. Pho, M.D., P.A.

Death by Food Pyramid: How Shoddy Science, Sketchy Politics and Shady Special Interests Ruined Your Health **by Denise Minger** is another book which is very revealing. Here is a brief description of the book on Amazon:

> "Warning: Shock and outrage will grip you as you dive into this one-of-a-kind exposé. Shoddy science, sketchy politics, and shady special interests have shaped American Dietary recommendations--and destroyed our nation's health--over recent decades. The phrase "death by food pyramid" isn't shock-value sensationalism, but the tragic consequence of following federal advice and corporate manipulation in pursuit of health.
>
> In Death by Food Pyramid, Denise Minger exposes the forces that overrode common sense and solid science to launch a pyramid phenomenon that bled far beyond US borders to taint the eating habits of the entire developed world"

Minger points out that the "experts," the "highly educated," and the "conventional wisdom" that promoted the idea that saturated fats will clog your arteries, and other misinformation are completely misguided. The consequences of following the "Food Pyramid" are dire at best.

> "… these guidelines might actually have had a negative impact on health, including our current obesity epidemic. [There's a] possibility that these dietary guidelines might actually be endangering health is at the core of our concern about the way guidelines are currently developed and issued."
>
> – Paul Marantz, Albert Einstein College of Medicine,
> *American Journal of Preventative Medicine*

Minger followed a vegetarian diet 80/10/10 with alarming consequences. She then goes on to tell the horrific story of the politicized food pyramid.

The Swedes were in need for cheaper food. Their focus was on cost rather than disease prevention. In attempt to help alleviate the high cost of food in Sweden, in 1974 Anna-Britt Agnsäter put together a food pyramid to visualize how to eat well but cut costs. At the base was dairy, grains, pasta and potatoes, in the middle was vegetables and fruits at the top was meat, fish and eggs. 20 years later the USDA came out with its infamous food pyramid which in many ways mirrored Agnsäter's pyramid.

You will find that some of the food groups will lead to a multitude of health issues. This has been proven by the statistics that show an enormous increase in obesity, diabetes and even new maladies of the brain which are on the increase. Based on the results, to follow the recommendations given by the establishment would be insane. You know what they say about insanity: "Insanity is doing the same thing over and over expecting different results."

"I diagnose by a clinical picture. I believe in clinical experience and clinical picture, much more than I believe in science. Our science has lost its way. ***More than 90% of scientific studies are commercially funded. They are deceptive.*** And the majority of us have no tools, and no training, to really decipher whether the study was designed properly, conducted properly, and then analyzed properly. It's very difficult. So there's a huge amount of information that leads you away from the truth. So I work with real people on a daily basis. I see what works and what doesn't work in real life. And if I need some scientific backing for any of those truths that I've discovered, I will find it. And usually those scientific studies are kosher… are correct. I believe in Mother Nature. I believe in real life, and real people." [**my emphasis**]

- Dr. Natasha Campbell-McBride
- *Gut-Brain Secrets, Good Food, Bad Food*

Following list is from a talk by Dr. Michael Eades author of *Protein Power*.
https://www.youtube.com/watch?v=wL5513xKw1k

- **1978** High Fructose Corn Syrup enters the market
- **1980** Obesity stable at 12-14% since 1960
  USDA releases low-fat guidelines
- **1984** NIH (National Institutes of Health)
  Lipid Research Clinic Study
  Anthony Gotto - President of AHA (American Heart Association)
  said "We will conquer atherosclerosis by the year 2000"
- **1986** NIH & AHA establish the NCEP (National Cholesterol
  Education Program) FDA says "no conclusive evidence" that sugar
  causes chronic disease
- **1987** Mevacor - first statin approved
- **1988** Surgeon General "**highest priority given to reducing fat in take**" C. Everett koop

Since the late 1970s, we have seen a huge increase in the number of diseases and those who have them. Obesity, diabetes, heart disease, stroke and new diseases of the brain are pandemic of biblical proportions. I believe this is a result of the recommendations of the various medical associations and bad science.

I went to the National Institutes of Health's website and copied what they said in 1988... **I disagree vehemently**!

> High intake of total dietary fat is associated with increased risk for obesity, some types of cancer, and possibly gallbladder disease. Epidemiological. clinical, and animal studies provide strong and consistent evidence for the relationship between saturated fat intake, high blood cholesterol, and increased risk for coronary heart-disease. Conversely, reducing blood cholesterol levels reduces the risk for death from coronary heart disease. Excessive saturated fat consumption is the major dietary contributor to total blood cholesterol levels. Dietary cholesterol raises blood cholesterol levels, but the effect is less pronounced than that of saturated fat. While polyunsaturated fatty acid consumption, and probably monounsaturated fatty acid consumption, lowers total blood cholesterol, the precise effects of specific fatty acids are not well defined. - NIH.gov - The Surgeon General's report on Nutrition and Health: Summary and Recommendations (1988)

If there was any evidence that the dietary guidelines were detrimental to our health, then the CDC's stats prove it was bad advice. The guidelines were introduced in 1980 at which point we see a dramatic increase in weight and obesity. Did we suddenly start eating more fat and cholesterol?

Was it butter, red meat, dairy? NO! The recommendation was eat low fat add grains, fruits, vegetable oils and eat less meat, eggs and dairy, which, for the most part, we did. Why did our ancestors before the 1900s not have an epidemic of heart disease, diabetes and other metabolic issues? Our ancestors ate meat, eggs and dairy.

"This [pharmaceutical] industry uses its wealth and power to co-opt every institution that might stand in its way, including the US Congress, the Food and Drug Administration, academic medical centers and the medical profession itself " - Dr. Marcia Angell, former editor of the New England Journal of Medicine - *The Truth about the Drug Companies: How They Deceive Us and What to Do about It.*

The USDA (United States Department of Agriculture) during this time (1980s) wanted to increase grain consumption. This goal could easily be reached if everyone followed the advice to eat a diet of low-fat and high carbohydrates. Since that time, we have seen an explosion of obesity and the related health problems.

"The main reason we take so many drugs is that drug companies don't sell drugs, they sell lies about drugs. This is what makes drugs so different from anything else in life...Virtually everything we know about drugs is what the companies have chosen to tell us and our doctors... the reason patients trust their medicine is that they extrapolate the trust they have in their doctors into the medicines they prescribe. The patients don't realize that, although their doctors may know a lot about diseases and human physiology and psychology, they know very, very little about drugs that hasn't been carefully concocted and dressed up by the drug industry.."

Deadly Medicines and Organized Crime - Peter Gotzsche

Statin Adverse Effects: A Review of the Literature and Evidence for a Mitochondrial Mechanism - Beatrice A. Golomb, M.D., Ph.D. and Marcella A. Evans - https://www.ncbi.nlm.nih.gov/pmc/articles/PMC2849981/

The following is a digest of: *Statin Adverse Effects (AEs) Supported by Evidence from Randomized Controlled Trials* (RCTs)

- Muscle - increase in myositis (inflammation of muscle)

- Cognition - Muscle and brain are classically affected in coenzyme-Q10-deficiency mitochondrial syndromes.

- Cancer - The sole randomized trial in the elderly (age >70) showed significant increase in incident cancer with statin use relative to placebo (HR 1.25, 95% CI 1.04-1.51, p=0.02)

- Liver - RCT data of LFT (liver function test) elevations are buttressed by many cases of statin hepatopathy (disorder of the liver)arising alone or in concert with statin rhabdomyolysis (potentially fatal disease that destroys skeletal muscle)

- Hemorrhagic Stroke - This extends evidence from observational data showing higher hemorrhagic stroke risk with low cholesterol

- Blood Glucose - High-dose statins led to statistically significant increase in glycemia in the PROVE-IT–TIMI trial

- Sleep - Also, there are case reports and case series of sleep problems and nightmares; and reports of sleep AEs in clinical trials of statins

"The AHA even rode the profit wave of refined carbohydrates from the 1990s onward by charging a hefty fee for the privilege of putting the AHA's "Heart Healthy" check mark on products, with the label ending up on some dubious candidates, such as Kellogg's Frosted Flakes, Fruity Marshmallow Krispies, and low-fat Pop-Tarts."
— Nina Teicholz, *The Big Fat Surprise: Why Meat, Butter, and Cheese Belong in a Healthy Diet*

Since the 1970s, we have successfully increased our fruits and vegetables by 17 percent, our grains by 29 percent, and reduced the amount of fat we eat from 43 percent to 33 percent of calories or less. The share of those fats that are saturated has also declined, according to the government's own data. (In these years, Americans also began exercising more.) Cutting back on fat has clearly meant eating more carbohydrates such as grains, rice, pasta, and fruit. A breakfast without eggs and bacon, for instance, is usually one of cereal or oatmeal; low-fat yogurt, a common breakfast choice, is higher in carbohydrates than the whole-fat version, because removing fat from foods nearly always requires adding carbohydrate-based "fat replacers" to make up for lost texture."
— Nina Teicholz, *The Big Fat Surprise: Why Meat, Butter, and Cheese Belong in a Healthy Diet*

Cholesterol and statins: Sham science and bad medicine

Michel de Lorgeril, M.D., is a cardiologist, nutritionist and researcher at France's National Center for Scientific Research (CNRS) and a member of the European Society of Cardiology

A description from his book on Amazon.com:

He speaks out against this collective regulatory insanity, based on biased, truncated and often falsified studies.

- The theory that cholesterol 'blocks arteries', that it causes heart attacks and strokes is an illusion that does not stand up to any physiological, experimental, epidemiological or clinical argument.

- Contrary to current dogma, statins do not reduce mortality, and this book provides irrefutable proof of this.

- These drugs, which can lead to diabetes and cancers, can also cause severe muscle damage, cognitive impairment and sexual dysfunction.

Doctors and patients need good quality scientific evidence in order to make informed decisions. But for decades now they have been misled by directives based on corrupt clinical studies, which have been knowingly altered to exaggerate the benefits of their molecules and to minimise their secondary effects. When their findings are carefully analyzed, nothing remains of their claims.

By far the most serious side effect, says Michel de Lorgeril, is that these prescriptions convey a false sense of security and prevent the population from adopting healthier lifestyle measures. Measures whose efficacy in the prevention of heart attacks and cardiovascular disease has been proven - and which are presented in this book

The Truth About the Drug Companies: How They Deceive Us and What to Do About It - Dr. Angell

(From a description of the book on Amazon)

During her two decades at "The "New England Journal of Medicine, Dr. Marcia Angell had a front-row seat on the appalling spectacle of the pharmaceutical industry. She watched drug companies stray from their original mission of discovering and manufacturing useful drugs and instead become vast marketing machines with unprecedented control over their own fortunes. She saw them gain nearly limitless influence over medical research, education, and how doctors do their jobs. She sympathized as the American public, particularly the elderly, struggled and increasingly failed to meet spiraling prescription drug prices. Now, in this bold, hard-hitting new book, Dr. Angell exposes the shocking truth of what the pharmaceutical industry has become-and argues for essential, long-overdue change.

Currently Americans spend a staggering $200 billion each year on prescription drugs. As Dr. Angell powerfully demonstrates, claims that high drug prices are necessary to fund research and development are unfounded: The truth is that drug companies funnel the bulk of their resources into the marketing of products of dubious benefit. Meanwhile, as profits soar, the companies brazenly use their wealth and power to push their agenda through Congress, the FDA, and academic medical centers.

Zeroing in on hugely successful drugs like AZT (the first drug to treat HIV/AIDS), Taxol (the best-selling cancer drug in history), and the blockbuster allergy drug Claritin, Dr. Angell demonstrates exactly how new products are brought to market. Drug companies, she shows, routinely rely on publicly funded institutions for their basic research; they rig clinical trials to make their products look better than they are; and they use their legions of lawyers to stretch out government-granted exclusive marketing rights for years. They also flood the market with copycat drugs that cost a lot more than the drugs they mimic but are no more effective.

The American pharmaceutical industry needs to be saved, mainly from itself, and Dr. Angell proposes a program of vital reforms, which includes restoring impartiality to clinical research and severing the ties between drug companies and medical education. Written with fierce passion and substantiated with in-depth research, "The Truth About the Drug Companies is a searing indictment of an industry that has spun out of control.

see also the video by Jack Bresler: *Swimming in Pills*:
https://vimeo.com/31058254

We are living in an age of deceit. It is getting more difficult to know who to trust. Many ads promise miraculous results, but are most times out and out fraud. If a product has a 30-day guarantee, and you get your money back, the benefit to them is they have had the use of your money for 30 days (a small interest free loan).

> "It is simply no longer possible to believe much of the clinical research that is published, or to rely on the judgment of trusted physicians or authoritative medical guidelines. I take no pleasure in this conclusion, which I reached slowly and reluctantly over my two decades as an editor of The New England Journal of Medicine." - Harvard Medical School's Dr. Marcia Angell

Drug companies distort the facts by trickery, promoting that their product will reduce the risk of death by some large percentage when, in fact, it is less than 2%. David Diamond points out that an ad for Lipitor® states that it will reduce the risk of fatal and non-fatal heart attacks by 36%. This is accomplished by dividing the factual risk when taking a placebo by the actual risk when taking the drug. In this case 98.1% did not die of a heart attack when taking the drug and 97% did not die when taking the placebo. The difference is 1.1%. Take the 1.1% difference and divide it by the 3%, and you get 36%. In reality, the only benefit of taking the statin over the placebo is minuscule, yet the ad falsely claims a much greater benefit.

Food companies proclaim that their food is healthy, and some even have the heart-healthy label even though it is full of empty carbohydrates and sugar. We have illustrated what happens when sugars and carbohydrates are processed by the body. Food companies try to say that all calories are the same, 100 calories in a can of soda is equivalent to 100 calories in a vegetable. This is provably false! Your body will disagree with that proposal. The body does not treat every calorie the same as we will illustrate!

AHA's (American Heart Association) income which is millions of dollars a year, comes from its "Heart-Check Certification Program." For a price, food companies, can pay to use the "Heart Healthy" symbol on their product, a red heart with a white check mark. The designation can be found on products which are NOT heart healthy, based on what we now know about sugar and carbohydrates.

> **Trust Us We're Experts: How Industry Manipulates Science and Gambles with Your Future - by John Stauber, Sheldon Rampton**
>
> "You think that nonprofit organizations just give away their stamps of approval on products? Bristol-Myers Squibb paid $600,000 to the American Heart Association for the right to display AHA's name and logo in ads for its cholesterol-lowering drug Pravachol. SmithKline Beecham paid the American Cancer Society $1 million for the right to use its logo in ads for Beecham's Nicoderm CQ and Nicorette anti-smoking ads.
>
> You think that if a scientist says so, it must be true? In the early 1990s, tobacco companies secretly paid thirteen scientists a total of $156,000 to write a few letters to influential medical journals. One biostatistician received $10,000 for writing a single, eight-paragraph letter that was published in the Journal of the American Medical Association. A cancer researcher received $20,137 for writing four letters and an opinion piece to the Lancet, the Journal of the National Cancer Institute, and The Wall Street Journal" (Quote from Amazon description of the book)

What about doctor error? I generally do not blame doctors, after all they are "practicing medicine." The human body is an extremely complex machine, knowing exactly how to deal with each instance is very difficult. Each one of us is distinct, our lifestyles, our backgrounds and our genetics. Sometimes doctors get it wrong, by outdated information from schooling, other times by faulty drug studies and often by guessing incorrectly.

Only medical doctors can prescribe drugs. The pharmaceutical companies spend enormous amounts of money promoting their products to doctors. However, have you noticed how many drugs are advertised in the media today? You are bombarded by ads touting the latest miracle drug, and you are innocently told to "ask your doctor" about drug X. There is a method to the madness. If enough people talk to their doctors about drug X, it is a silent promotion of their product to doctors. "Word of mouth works!"

See the book *The Big Fix: How The Pharmaceutical Industry Rips Off American Consumers (Public-affairs Reports)* by Katharine Greider

At the time I am writing this you can read a report by Dr. Gary Null M.D., which documents the issues and cost of misdiagnoses in terms of money and lives:
www.newmediaexplorer.org/sepp/Death by Medicine Nov 27.doc

From the **bmj** (the British Medical Journal:)

Big pharma often commits corporate crime, and this must be stopped BMJ 2012; 345 doi: https://doi.org/10.1136/bmj.e8462 (Published 14 December 2012) BMJ 2012;345:e8462

Peter C Gøtzsche, professor, Nordic Cochrane Centre, Rigshospitalet, Blegdamsvej

When a drug company commits a serious crime, the standard response from the industry is that there are bad apples in any enterprise. Sure, but the interesting question is whether drug companies routinely break the law.

I googled the names of the 10 largest drug companies in combination with the term "fraud" and looked for offenses on the first page for each company. The most common recent crimes were illegal marketing by recommending drugs for non-approved (off label) uses, misrepresentation of research results, hiding data on harms, and Medicaid and Medicare fraud.1 All cases were related to the United States and involved huge settlements or fines, exceeding $1bn (£620.6m; €769m) each for four companies.

It was easy to find additional crimes committed by these same companies and committed outside the US. As the crimes were widespread and repetitive, they are probably committed deliberately—because crime pays. Pfizer, for example, agreed in 2009 to pay $430m to resolve charges related to illegal marketing of gabapentin (Neurontin), but as sales were $2.7bn in 2003 alone, and as about 90% was for off label use...

> "For a modern disease to be related to an old fashioned food (e.g. red meat) is one of the most ludicrous things I have ever heard in my life"
> - Peter Cleave, Surgeon Captain (1906-1983)
>
> "We have a multi-billion dollar industry that is killing people, right and left, just for financial gain. Their idea of research is to see whether two doses of this poison is better than three doses of that poison."
> — Dr. Glenn A. Warner, M.D. (1919-2000).

> "The combined profits for the ten drug companies in the Fortune 500 ($35.9 billion) were more than the profits for all the other 490 businesses put together ($33.7 billion) [in 2002]. Over the past two decades the pharmaceutical industry has moved very far from its original high purpose of discovering and producing useful new drugs. Now primarily a marketing machine to sell drugs of dubious benefit, this industry uses its wealth and power to co-opt every institution that might stand in its way, including the US Congress, the FDA, academic medical centers, and the medical profession itself." - Dr. Marcia Angell - *The Truth About the Drug Companies* - Dr. Angell is a former editor in chief of the prestigious New England Journal of Medicine.

Ellen G. White and the Seventh Day Adventist:

In 1938 the Seventh-Day Adventists put Ellen G. White's writings on health in a book titled *Counsels on Diets and Foods.* The following are a few quotes from that book:

"Meat should not be placed before our children. Its influence is to excite and strengthen the lower passions, and has a tendency to deaden the moral powers. Grains and fruits prepared free from grease, and in as natural a condition as possible, should be the food for the tables of all who claim to be preparing for translation to heaven." (pp. 63-64)

"They [parents] tempt their children to indulge their appetite by placing upon their tables flesh meats and other food prepared with spices, which have a tendency to excite the animal passions." (pp. 231-232)

"Vegetables, fruits, and grains should compose our diet. Not an ounce of flesh meat should enter our stomachs. The eating of flesh is unnatural. We are to return to God's original purpose in the creation of man." (p. 380)

"Among those who are waiting for the coming of the Lord, meat eating will eventually be done away: flesh will cease to form a part of their diet." p. 380.

"It has been clearly presented to me that God's people are to take a firm stand against meat eating." (p. 383)

"But since the Lord presented before me, in June, 1863, the subject of meat eating in relation to health, I have left the use of meat. For a while it was rather difficult to bring my appetite to bread, for which, formerly, I had but little relish. But by persevering, I have been able to do this. I have lived for nearly one year without meat. For about six months most of the bread upon our table has been unleavened cakes, made of unbolted wheat meal and water, and a very little salt. We use fruits and vegetables liberally. I have lived for eight months upon two meals a day." p. 482.

"The health reform, I was shown, is a part of the third angel's message and is just as closely connected with it as are the arm and hand with the human body." p.486.

White believed in a strict vegetarian diet and the Seventh-Day Adventists still hold to that today.

John Harvey Kellogg

John Harvey Kellogg in the 19th century during a time when sexuality was frowned on especially masturbation had very definite feelings about sex. "Self-pollution is a crime doubly abominable."

Like Ellen G. White, Kellogg thought that meat and certain foods increased sexual desire. Kellogg was a strict vegetarian and follower of the Seventh-Day Adventist diet and an active member. While working as superintendent at Michigan's Battle Creek Sanitarium, he tried a few different "healthy" eating concoctions using oatmeal and corn in 1878. He invented corn flakes, which were touted as healthy and ready-to-eat. Of course, cornflakes were never advertised and there is doubt that he invented Corn Flakes as a way to curb masturbation. However, his strong beliefs would lead us to believe that it may have something to do with sexuality. Like his quote:

"The influence of coffee in stimulating the genital organs is notorious"
— John Harvey Kellogg

We have revealed throughout this book that saturated fats and cholestrol are not the main cause of heart disease. It was later discovered that Hegsted's research had been funded by the sugar industry. Hegsted was critical of the idea that sugar consumption was the cause of heart disease, something we now know is untrue. However, because of Hegsted's credentials his theories were given credence and accepted by the McGovern committee.

Dr. Robert Levy, National Heart Lung and Blood Institute director stated during the hearings:

> "With cholesterol the issue is a little more murky. We have no doubt from the vast amount of epidemiological data available that elevated [blood] cholesterol is associated with an increased risk of heart attack, especially some specific types of … cholesterol. We have no doubt that cholesterol can be lowered by diet, and/or medication in most patients. **Where the doubt exists is the question of whether lowering cholesterol will result in a reduced incidence of heart attack; that is still presumptive**. It is unproven [in clinical trials], but **there is a tremendous amount of circumstantial evidence**…. There is no doubt that cholesterol can be lowered by diet in free living populations. It can be lowered by 10 to 15 percent. **The problem with all these trials is that none of them have showed a difference in heart attack or death rate in the treated group**." (my emphasis)

It is clear that Dr. Levy had serious doubts about the question of the lipid hypothesis and disease. In the final analysis, the committee bent to special interest groups and political contentions. This is often the cause of many government programs gone astray ending in actually harming the public it is tasked with helping. During this time (1977) there was a rush to complete the task of the McGovern committee and McGovern said:

> "Senators do not have the luxury that the research scientist does of waiting until every last shred of evidence is in,"

This rush to judgment has caused an unlimited amount of pain and suffering to the majority of those who followed their ill-advised nutritional advice as witnessed by the increase in ill-health and disease.

You read the details of the of this committee at:
https://www.ncbi.nlm.nih.gov/pmc/articles/PMC3910043/

When the government gets involved in controlling outcomes, disaster is right around the corner. We could give numerous examples of how things actually get worse when the government tries to "fix" things. For our purposes here we will focus on the infamous: *McGovern's Senate Select Committee on Nutrition and Human Needs.* It began with a desire to wipe out under-nutrition. In 1968 after a CBS documentary, *Hunger in America*, revealed that too many Americans were suffering from under-nutrition.

> "The idea that people were going hungry in the land of plenty ... elicited widespread demands for expansion of federal food assistance programs."
>
> - G. McGovern, Statement of Senator George McGovern on the Publication of Dietary Goals for the United States, Press Conference, Friday, February 14, 1977, in United States Senate Select Committee on Nutrition and Human Needs, Dietary Goals for the United States (Washington, DC: US Government Printing Office, February 1977)

Often good intentions end up making a bad situation even worse. And like every government program once started, they are almost impossible to reverse. As a result, we find ourselves with increasing obesity and many diseases, which eventually cause serious injury or kill as a result of the McGovern committee's recommendations.

David Mark Hegsted was one of those who testified during the McGovern committee meetings. Hegsted had studied the connection of food consumption and heart disease.

> "The equation he developed showed that cholesterol and saturated fats from sources such as eggs and meat in the diet raised harmful cholesterol levels, mono-unsaturated fats had little effect and polyunsaturated fats from sources such as nuts and seeds lowered levels. Results from these studies were published in 1965 in the American Journal of Clinical Nutrition, to what was described by The New York Times as "great acclaim". In combination with research performed independently by Ancel Keys, these results led to recommendations advocating decreased dietary consumption of saturated fats. - Jeremy Pearce "*D. Mark Hegsted, 95, Harvard Nutritionist, Is Dead*", The New York Times, July 8, 2009.

The Root Cause in the dramatic rise of Chronic Disease

What has happened since we followed the advice from the McGovern commission in the late 1970s?

Autism (2,094%)	*Alzheimer's* (299%)
COPD (148%)	**diabetes (305%)**
Sleep apnea (430%)	celiac disease (1,111%)
ADHD (819%)	asthma (142%)
Depression (280%)	*youth bipolar disease* (10,833%)
Osteoarthritis (449%)	lupus (787%)
Inflammatory bowel (120%)	chronic fatigue (11,027%)
fibromyalgia (7,727%)	multiple sclerosis (117%)
hypothyroidism (702%)."	

According to the article Richard Lear attributes the increase in disease to peroxynitrite. Peroxynitrite is formed when l-arginine (an amino acid) is not converted to nitric oxide (NO). This conversion causes inflammation setting off a cascade of events causing the death of the mitochondria. When superoxide and nitric oxide radicals exist simultaneously in the cell trouble begins; necrosis or apoptosis of the cell will be the outcome. All of the above diseases have been associated with peroxynitrite. If you want a detailed scientific explanation see:

https://www.sciencedirect.com/topics/pharmacology-toxicology-and-pharmaceutical-science/peroxynitrite

The mitochondria are responsible for many functions; energy production, calcium homeostasis and the creation of new complex molecules out of simpler, smaller precursors (known as the biosynthesis pathway). Mitochondrial dysfunction is associated with many diseases; diabetes, stroke, atherosclerosis and many others. It is my hope that you see that health is a very complex subject, one we could not begin to address in any great detail in this book.

"...It does not require a majority to prevail, but rather an irate, tireless minority keen to set brush fires in people's minds.."

-Samuel Adams

XII

FINAL THOUGHTS

If you have any of the issues we talked about, and you have learned anything from this book, then, please contact one of the medical professionals or research the issues from the resources in appendix B and get the help you need before it is too late. What have you got to lose?

Today, deception is in full force in the areas of health, science and politics. The method of attack is to discredit the opposition or to state that the idea has been established and cannot be debated. I could quote several times when I heard that phrase "it is not debatable." Example Harry Reid, Senate Democrat leader at the time said, "Global warming is not debatable." They will refuse to debate the relevant issues and *cover up* opposing points of view. However, this technique is used to promote other issues: socialism, global warming, and other hot issues. This book is about the lies and deception of the lipid hypothesis and current medical practice.

> If you tell a lie big enough and keep repeating it, people will eventually come to believe it. The lie can be maintained only for such time as the State can shield the people from the political, economic and/or military consequences of the lie. It thus becomes vitally important for the State to use all of its powers to repress dissent, for the truth is the mortal enemy of the lie, and thus by extension, the truth is the greatest enemy of the State.
>
> Joseph Goebbels quotes - of the Third Reich

It is obvious to me, but may not be to others. We are designed in a very specific way. Our bodies are complex beyond our comprehension! We have observed in our discussion that the food, drug and medical profession have bamboozled us with misleading and sometimes fraudulent information. Some in the profession automatically accept what the so-called "experts," tell them; others are not open to anything but the commonly accepted views and are afraid of change. This causes the ideas to be "locked in stone" and perpetuated for years to come. Once these ideas are accepted and passed on as absolute fact, and repeated, it is virtually impossible to change minds. This is generally the result of pride and arrogance by those who promote their ideas either based on willing ignorance or by financial gains, they get from the industry.

Ask anyone on the street if high cholesterol causes heart disease, and they will tell you emphatically that it does. Does saturated fat cause you to get fat and develop heart problems, again the answer will come back loud and clear, YES! I believe that we have illustrated that we have been deceived into believing the lie. The evidence is clearly before us; a dramatic increase in obesity, and a multitude of diseases because we follow the advice of the experts!

Official science: The grand illusion

Posted on January 15, 2016 - PersonalLiberty.com

"Government science exists because it is a fine weapon to use, in order to force an agenda of control over the population. We aren't talking about knowledge here. Knowledge is irrelevant. What counts is: 'How can we fabricate something that looks like the truth?' I keep pointing this out: we're dealing with reality builders. In this case, they make their roads and fences out of data, and they massage and invent the data out of thin air to suit their purposes. After all, they also invent money out of thin air."

— *"The Underground"* by Jon Rappoport
    http://www.nomorefakenews.com/

Now I want to switch gears and tell you that belief in evolution or the statement that "we adapted" is every bit as unwise as following the advice of the food, drug and educational institutions. It has been ingrained in the fabric of our culture, and it is wrong. I only ask that you research for yourself how ridiculous that belief is to anyone who will take the time to study it without bias. You don't have to believe me check out the video on youtube at: https://www.youtube.com/watch?v=noj4phMT9OE
with David Berlinsky, Stephen Meyer and David Gelernter.

An article in the Claremont Review of Books by David Gelernter a professor of computer science at Yale University called *Giving up Darwin*, explains mathematically how Darwin's theory of origins is not plausible.

If you take the totality of all the functions and intricate inter-dependabilities of the human body, and the fact that all of these must exist all at the same time Darwin's idea falls apart. Can you exist without ATP or without the Sodium/Potassium pumps or how about a complete and operational immune system? I could go on naming systems, chemical interactions, immune facilities and hormones that must all be present at the same time and what about homeostasis? How would undirected chance have the information (knowledge) to know what is required to keep us in balance? Temperature, blood sugar levels, and a host of other balances? If any of these complex systems were not in existence at the same time, then you cease to exist in a very short time. Many do cease to exist today when these intricate systems begin to fail because of poor diet, environmental issues and the stress of daily living. And how would all of the chemicals and processes come about by chance. I don't care how much time you have; you could not evolve because you would cease to exist before you could get started. It is a chicken and egg problem. Which came first DNA or amino acids?

> "There is no reason to doubt that Darwin successfully explained the small adjustment by which an organism adapts to local circumstances: changes to fur density or wing style or beak shape. Yet there are many reasons to doubt whether he can explain the big picture — not the fine-tuning of species but the emergence of new ones."
>
> David Gelernter, *Giving Up Darwinism - Claremont Review of Books*

Dr. Dean Kenyon co-authored a book called <u>*Biochemical Predestination,*</u> in this book he put forth the idea that biochemical molecular compounds such as proteins, could assemble themselves from non-living raw chemicals given the right environmental conditions. This book is still used in universities today to prove evolution. However, Dr. Kenyon recanted his hypothesis, because the theory of biochemical predestination fails to explain how complex amino acid based proteins self assemble without or prior to, the existence of DNA based sequencing or assembly codes. Dr.

Kenyon is a rare example of clear unbiased thinking. To admit that his hypothesis was incorrect, after gaining such notoriety, is truly the mark of a great man.

"Since molecular biologists began to appreciate the sequence specificity of proteins and nucleic acids, many calculations have been made to determine the probability of formulating functional proteins and nucleic acids at random. … Such calculations have invariably shown that the probability of obtaining functionally sequenced biomacromolecules at random is, in [Nobelist Ilya] Prigogine's words, 'vanishingly small'. … Chance is not an adequate explanation for the origin of biological complexity and specificity."
- Stephen C. Meyer,
The Message in the Microcosm: DNA and the Death of Materialism," Cosmic Pursuit, Fall 1997.

To quote Darwin himself:

> "If it could be demonstrated that any complex organ existed, which could not possibly have been formed by numerous, successive, slight modifications, my theory would absolutely break down." - Darwin

"A Lie doesn't become truth, wrong doesn't become right and evil doesn't become good, just because it's accepted by a majority."
— Booker T. Washington

Darwin had no knowledge of DNA or a host of other systems in the human body. What he did not know would fill volumes of books. If Darwin put forth his idea today, knowing all that we now know, would he be taken seriously? I doubt it. However, once an idea is accepted it takes a long time to undo the damage cause by the erroneous information, we have seen this in the saturated fat is bad prognosis. This misinformation is then passed on generation after generation until it is ingrained in the minds as fact.

Science now knows that many of the pillars of Darwinian theory are either false Or misleading. Yet biology texts continue to present them as factual evidence of Evolution. What does this imply about their scientific standards?
— Jonathan wells

Final Thoughts ▬▬▬▬▬▬▬▬▬▬▬▬▬▬▬▬▬▬▬▬▬▬▬▬▬▬▬▬▬▬

In this case, it is a desire to keep a designer out of the picture by perpetuating the lie. This is parallel to what is happening in the health industry and how they explain what is the underlying cause of disease, it is how they continue to propagate false ideas.

"It is not that the methods and institutions of science somehow compel us to accept a material explanation of the phenomenal world, but, on the contrary, that we are forced by our **a priori*** adherence to material causes to create an apparatus of investigation and a set of concepts that produce material explanations, no matter how counter-intuitive, no matter how mystifying to the uninitiated. Moreover, that materialism is absolute, for we cannot allow a **Divine Foot in the door.**" - Richard C. Lewontin and Thomas Nagel Living organisms "appear to have been carefully and artfully designed." [my emphasis]

definition of **a priori from the Web: involving deductive reasoning from a general principle to a necessary effect; not supported by fact; "as a priori judgment"*

"In each cell (humans have about 300 trillion) "there are multiple operating systems, multiple programming languages, encoding/decoding hardware and software, specialized communications systems, error detection and correction mechanisms, specialized input/output channels for organelle control and feedback, and a variety of specialized 'devices' to accomplish the tasks of life... The challenge for an undirected origin of such a cybernetic complex interacting computer system is the need to demonstrate that the rules, laws, and theories that govern electronic computing systems and information don't apply to the even more complex digital information systems that are in living organisms. Laws of chemistry and physics, which follow exact statistical, thermodynamic, and spacial laws, are totally inadequate for generating complex functional information or those systems that process that information using prescriptive algorithmic information." *Probability's Nature & Natures Probability -A Call to Scientific Integrity* (p. 47) - Dr. Donald E. Johnson

It is not my intent to convince you that Darwin was wrong, only to hopefully prick your interest enough to check it out for yourself and not be like the masses that take something as true which has not be proven.

> To grasp the reality of life as it has been revealed by molecular biology, we must magnify a cell a thousand million times until it is twenty kilometers in diameter and resembles a giant airship large enough to cover a great city like London or New York. What we would then see would be an object of unparalleled complexity and adaptive design. On the surface of the cell we would see millions of openings, like the port holes of a vast space ship, opening and closing to allow a continual stream of materials to flow in and out. If we were to enter one of these openings we would find ourselves in a world of supreme technology and bewildering complexity... Is it really credible that random processes could have constructed a reality, the smallest element of which-a functional protein or gene-is complex beyond our own creative capacities, a reality which is the very antithesis of chance, which excels in every sense anything produced by the intelligence of man?
>
> Michael Denton, *Evolution: A Theory in Crisis*, Burnett Books, London, 1985, pp. 328, 342.

Think for just a moment, if undirected evolution were true then, how would male and female evolve and be such a perfect match for procreation without a designer? First, if you think evolution was accomplished by mutations over millions of years, try again mutations are virtually NEVER an improvement. Even if it were possible, the DNA must change for the next generation to maintain the improvements. How would that happen?

Undirected chance mutations _can never_ anticipate future problems that may arise in its environment! Natural Selection takes place after the fact so it is no help. ONLY a designer would know how to build in contingencies! We could name hundreds of things that must deal with these contingencies. Without these built-in contingencies the organism would die and that would end the process of evolution. One example is the blood clotting cascade. How could undirected chance mutations anticipate the need to stop blood flow and only at the source of the wound? Trial and error in this very complex process will most certainly eliminate the organism immediately upon the first cut! (for more detail see my book *The Body Map - Designed from the Beginning*.)

"Many evolutionary propagandists are guilty of the deceitful practice of equivocation, that is, switching the meaning of a single word (evolution) part way through an argument. A common tactic, 'bait-and-switch,' is simply to produce examples of change over time, call this 'evolution,' then imply that the GTE [General Theory of Evolution] is thereby proven or even essential, and creation disproved. The PBS Evolution series and the Scientific American article are full of examples of this fallacy". ─ Jonathan Sarfati,Ph.D., F.M. *Refuting Evolution 2*,

I.L. Cohen makes a good point, that there is a very fine balance in the DNA. To upset this balance does not bring about positive effects.

"Summing it up, and contrary to the oft-repeated evolutionist claims, a random mutation is not an enhancing factor -- it is almost invariably a destructive one. It interferes with the exquisitely fine balance and purposefulness of the hundreds of millions of nucleotides within a given program. To propose and argue that mutations even in tandem with 'natural selection' are the root-causes for 6,000,000 viable, enormously complex species, is to mock logic, deny the weight of evidence, and reject the fundamentals of mathematical probability." ˉ Cohen, I.L. *In Darwin Was Wrong - A Study in Probabilities*.
New Research Publications, Inc., New York, NY (1984), p.81.

Biologist Ranganathan agrees that changes in a highly ordered system do not make a system better.

"Genuine mutations are very rare in nature. Most mutations are harmful since they are random, rather than orderly changes in the structure of genes; any random change in a highly ordered system will be for the worse, not for the better. For example, if an earthquake were to shake a highly ordered structure such as a building, there would be a random change in the framework of the building, which, in all probability, would not be an improvement." . G. Ranganathan, *Origins?, Pennsylvania: The Banner Of Truth Trust, 1988*

"There is no chance ($<10^{-1000}$) to see this mechanism appear spontaneously and if it did, even less for it to remain."

- Marcel P. Schutzenberger
Algorithms and the Neo-Darwinian Theory of Evolution

We look at an airplane and marvel at its design and function, then turn around look at the magnificent design of the human body. Just comparing those two, no one would believe an airplane was accidentally formed, and yet today's evolutionary scientists would have us believe that everything we see was the result of a series of accidents. This is insane! I do not believe that even Darwin, if he had known the things that we now know, would have dared suggest that accidental blind chance could ever have structured what we see today. Even at that, he did express concern on how sight could be developed with slight modifications.

Some beliefs are passed on without a thorough examination of the facts. Just like the statements "eggs, dairy, red meat and saturated fat are bad" these ideas have been passed on for decades now, and they are dead wrong. Accepting evolution as fact when common sense tells you how impossible it would be is equally as wrong. Although, just like the food and drug industries, they have a vested interest in maintaining status quo, belief in evolution has its own collaborators wanting to keep the existence of a creator out of the minds of us all. Evolutionists, the Food/drug industry and the medical profession will fight to the death to maintain their long-held beliefs no matter who it effects... or harms. That is a sad reality!

Editorial from the BMJ:

Saturated fat **<u>does not</u>** clog the arteries: coronary heart disease is a chronic inflammatory condition, the risk of which can be effectively reduced from healthy lifestyle interventions - Aseem Malhotra, Rita F Redberg, Pascal Meier...

Appendix A

Tables and Graphs

Tables & Graphs

The following is a list of sugars you may encounter in your food:

agave nectar	barley malt	blackstrap molasses
brown rice syrup	brown sugar	coconut
sugar		
cane sugar	corn syrup	date sugar
dextrin	diastatic malt	dextrose
ethyl maltol	florida crystals	fructose
fruit juice	glucose	golden syrup
high-fructose corn syrup	honey	lactose
levulose	maltodextrin	muscovado
maltose	maple sugar	molasses
nonfat dry milk	palm sugar	panocha
sorgum syurp	sorbitol	saccharose
skimmed milk	powder sorghum	sucrose
treacle	turbinado	

Fatty Acid Profiles of Common Fats & Oils

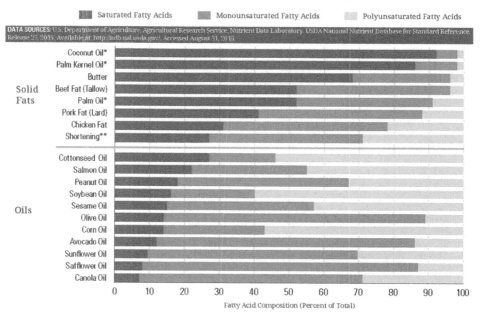

Fatty Acid Composition (Percent of Total)

From the website: https://www.msgmyth.com/hidden-names used with permission. The following substances always contain factory created free glutamate, with MSG containing 78%.

MSG
Mono sodium glutamate
Mono potassium glutamate
Glutamate
Glutamic Acid
Vegetable Protein Extract
Calcium Caseinate
Mono ammonium glutamate
Natrium glutamate
Anything hydrolyzed or autolyzed

Gelatin
Hydrolyzed Vegetable Protein
Hydrolyzed Plant Protein (HPP)
Autolyzed Plant Protein
Sodium Caseinate
Senomyx (labeled:artificial flavor)
Sodium caseinate
Soy protein,
Ajinomoto

Calcium glutamate
Textured Protein
Yeast Extract
Yeast food or nutrient
Autolyzed Yeast
Any hydrolyzed protein
Magnesium glutamate
Whey protein, whey protein isolate
Vestin

BOOK: *Battling the MSG Myth* - by Debby Anglesey

Autism (2,094%)   *Alzheimer's* (299%)
COPD (148%)   **diabetes (305%)**
Sleep apnea (430%)   celiac disease (1,111%)
ADHD (819%)   asthma (142%)
Depression (280%)   *youth bipolar disease* (10,833%)
Osteoarthritis (449%)   lupus (787%)
Inflammatory bowel (120%)   chronic fatigue (11,027%)
fibromyalgia (7,727%)   multiple sclerosis (117%)
hypothyroidism (702%)."

Sources of Lectins:

Soy beans	kidney beans	navy beans
pinto beans	lima Beans	lava beans
wax beans	Castor beans	jack beans
string beans	Sweet peas	green peas
cow peas	horse grams	barley
corn	rice	wheat
wheat germ	tomatoes	potatoes
sweet potatoes	zucchini	carrots
rhubarb	beets	mushrooms
asparagus	turnips	cucumbers
pumpkin	sweet peppers	radishes
oranges	lemons	grapefruit
blackberries	raspberries	strawberries.
pomegranate	grapes	cherries
quinces	apples	watermelon
banana	papaya	plums
currants	Walnuts	hazelnuts
peanuts	sunflower seeds	sesame seeds
coconut	chocolate	coffee
caraway	nutmeg	peppermint
marjoram	garlic	egg plant

Cornell University: Plant Lectins

Food Guide Pyramid
A Guide to Daily Food Choices

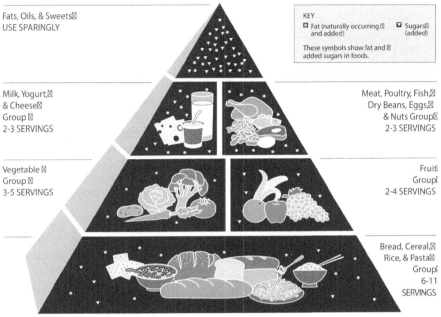

Fats, Oils, & Sweets
USE SPARINGLY

KEY
▢ Fat (naturally occurring   ▨ Sugars
  and added)   (added)
These symbols show fat and
added sugars in foods.

Milk, Yogurt,
& Cheese
Group
2-3 SERVINGS

Meat, Poultry, Fish,
Dry Beans, Eggs,
& Nuts Group
2-3 SERVINGS

Vegetable
Group
3-5 SERVINGS

Fruit
Group
2-4 SERVINGS

Bread, Cereal,
Rice, & Pasta
Group
6-11
SERVINGS

Source: U.S. Department of Agriculture/U.S. Department of Health and Human Services

The Endrocrine System
HORMONES

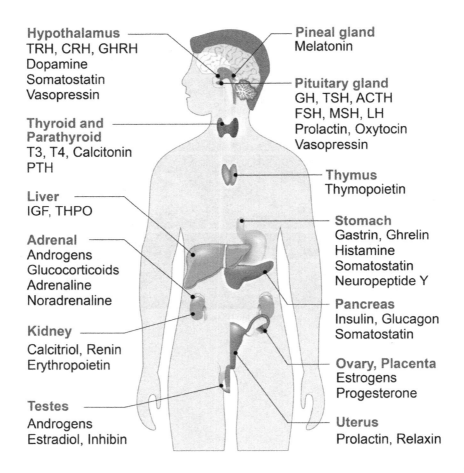

Hypothalamus
TRH, CRH, GHRH
Dopamine
Somatostatin
Vasopressin

Thyroid and Parathyroid
T3, T4, Calcitonin
PTH

Liver
IGF, THPO

Adrenal
Androgens
Glucocorticoids
Adrenaline
Noradrenaline

Kidney
Calcitriol, Renin
Erythropoietin

Testes
Androgens
Estradiol, Inhibin

Pineal gland
Melatonin

Pituitary gland
GH, TSH, ACTH
FSH, MSH, LH
Prolactin, Oxytocin
Vasopressin

Thymus
Thymopoietin

Stomach
Gastrin, Ghrelin
Histamine
Somatostatin
Neuropeptide Y

Pancreas
Insulin, Glucagon
Somatostatin

Ovary, Placenta
Estrogens
Progesterone

Uterus
Prolactin, Relaxin

How do the cells get energy from food?

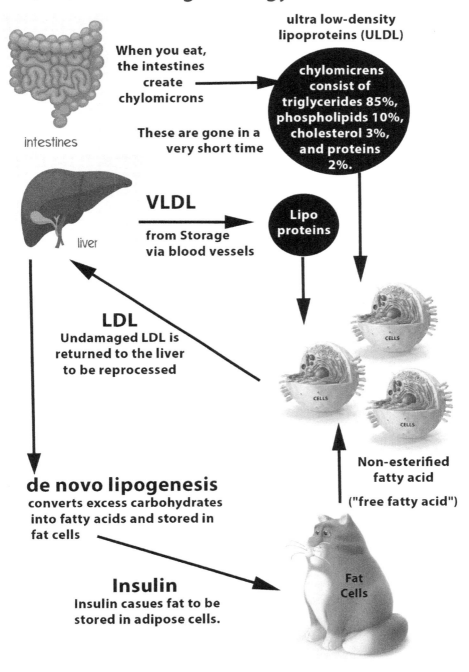

ultra low-density
lipoproteins (ULDL)

When you eat,
the intestines
create
chylomicrons

chylomicrens
consist of
triglycerides 85%,
phospholipids 10%,
cholesterol 3%,
and proteins
2%.

These are gone in a
very short time

intestines

VLDL

from Storage
via blood vessels

Lipo
proteins

liver

LDL
Undamaged LDL is
returned to the liver
to be reprocessed

CELLS

CELLS

CELLS

Non-esterified
fatty acid

("free fatty acid")

de novo lipogenesis
converts excess carbohydrates
into fatty acids and stored in
fat cells

Insulin
Insulin casues fat to be
stored in adipose cells.

Fat
Cells

Signs and symptoms of
Hypothyroidism

Psychological
- Poor memory and
  concentration

- Poor hearing

Pharynx
- Hoarseness

Heart
- Slow pulse rate
- Pericardial effusion

Muscular
- Delayed reflex
  relaxation

Extremities
- Coldness
- Carpal tunnel
  syndrome

General
- Fatigue
- Feeling cold
- Weight gain with
  poor appetite

- Hair loss

Lungs
- Shortness of breath
- Pleural effusion

Skin
- Paresthesia
- Myxedema

Intestines
- Constipation
- Ascites

*Reproductive
system*
- Menorrhagia

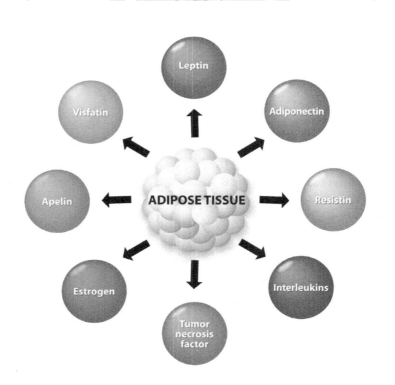

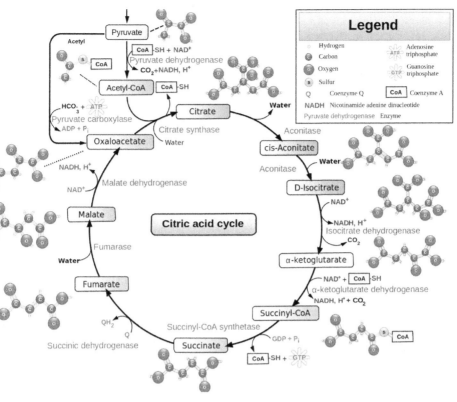

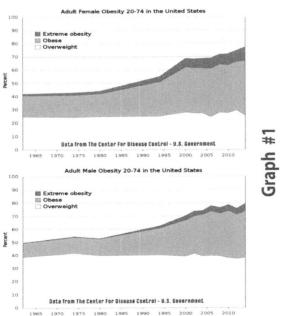

Graph #1

STAGES OF ATHEROSCLEROSIS

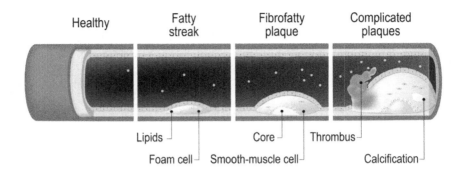

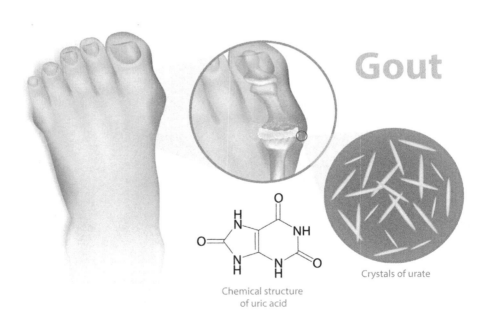

Chemical structure of uric acid

Crystals of urate

During Increased activity in a muscle cell.

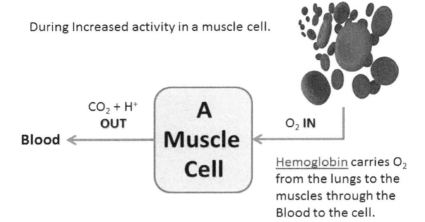

$CO_2 + H^+$
OUT

A Muscle Cell

Blood ←

O_2 **IN**

Hemoglobin carries O_2 from the lungs to the muscles through the Blood to the cell.

Appendix B

Glossary of Terms

Acidosis - an increase of acidity in the blood.

ADHD (819% increase since the 1980s) - Attention deficit hyperactivity disorder - problems in paying attention, excessive activity.

Adipose - are fat cells. You have likely heard about white fat and brown fat. White fat is used for the storage of energy and brown fat generates body heat. However, you can have too much white fat. The obese have an excess adipose tissue. Even then there is different places where this fat cells reside: subcutaneous under the skin, visceral fat around the organs (liver, kidneys, etc.), Epicardial around the heart

Adipogenesis - the production of fat or depositing of fat in the cell. It is also the conversion of carbohydrates or protein to fat.

AGEs - advanced glycation end products generate free radicals and the oxidation of LDL. Oxidized LDL is the type of cholesterol which collects in the arteries. White blood cells are tasked with destroying them but doesn't always accomplish the task. The level of AGEs in the blood can indicate the possibility of coronary heart disease. AGEs can also cause changes which damage the filtering segments of the kidneys.

Alzheimer's (299% increase since the 1980s) a progressive disease which gets worse over time and symptoms are: disorientation, mood swings, trouble remembering people and events.

Alanine aminotransferase, (ALT)
Enzymes that break down proteins to allow the body to digest them. If the body is damaged you may find ALT in the blood steam indicating liver damage.

Amyotrophic lateral sclerosis (ALS) - also known as Lou Gehrig's Disease, this aliment causes the death of neurons in the brain which control voluntary muscles. Also ALS is a nerve destroying, muscle wasting condition.

Androgen - (from Greek andr meaning male) hormones testosterone and Dihydrotestosterone (DHT) are androgens.

Apolipoprotein B - the total number of LDL lipoprotein particles

Apoptosis - Programmed cell death, a process where cells are deliberately and systematically killed off. It is a necessary part of healthy cell function. When apoptosis is hindered by some mechanism cancers is the outcome.

Asthma (142%) - an inflammatory disease blocking the airways of the lungs. Symptoms: shortness of breath, wheezing, chest tightness.

Atherogenic dyslipidemia - a condition where there is a high level of LDL and triglycerides and a low level of HDL.

ATP (see mitochondria)

Autism (2094% since the 1980s) extreme trouble with social interaction

Autoimmune - when the immune system starts attacking the body's own healthy tissue.

Autophagy (a-tof i-gee) - meaning "self-devouring" a process where by the unnecessary or dysfunctional cellular components are recycled or removed.

B-hydroxybutrate - A keytone body that acts as an energy source. BHB is especially efficient in providing energy for the brain and can release neurotrophins. The keytones reduce the production of ROS or reactive oxygen species in addition to a clean up function or ROS by other processes.

Beta-amyloid plaque - a brain chemical associated with Alzheimer's and other maladies.
"Similar plaques appear in some variants of Lewy body dementia and in inclusion body myositis (a muscle disease), while Aβ can also form the aggregates that coat cerebral blood vessels in cerebral amyloid angiopathy. The plaques are composed of a tangle of regularly ordered fibrillar aggregates called amyloid fibers" - Parker MH, Reitz AB (2000). *"Assembly of β-Amyloid Aggregates at the Molecular Level"*. Chemtracts-Organic Chemistry. 13 (1): 51–56.

Bipolar disease – youth (10,833% increase since the 1980s) a mental disorder switching from depression to elevated moods.

Glossary of Terms

Body Mass Index (BMI)—A measure of weight in kilograms (kg) relative to height in meters squared (m2). BMI is considered a reasonably reliable indicator of total body fat, which is related to the risk of disease and death. - USDA.gov

Blood Pressure Homeostasis: Low blood pressure is called hypotension and can be caused by things like dehydration and lose blood from a major cut. Hypotension, if not corrected, can cause fainting or worse, kidney failure. Hypertension occurs when the blood pressure is too high and can ultimately, if not brought into balance, cause a stroke.

There are two hormones which affect the cardiovascular system, ADH (anti-diuretic hormone - stimulates contraction of arteries and capillaries) and epinephrine (known as adrenaline).

The baroreceptor (baro means pressure) found in the carotid sinuses (blood which is going to the brain) and the aortic arch (blood going to the body) are receptors. These receptors communicate to the brain changes in **the stretch,** in the veins. The brain remembers what your normal set point is, say 120/80 because of the number of action potentials it receives through the central nervous system. If that number goes up, the brain knows that blood pressure is above normal. If the number of action potentials goes down, then the brain knows that blood pressure is dropping.

There are two nervous system inputs to the heart, sympathetic input and parasympathetic. Sympathetic will increase the heart rate pumping more blood and parasympathetic input will decrease the rate.

Additionally, endothelial receptors control the restriction of blood vessels. These receptors are found in the smooth muscle tissue of blood vessels. Endothelins attempt to maintain a balance between vasoconstriction (constriction) and vasodilation. (Dilation) of blood vessels.

Celiac disease (1111% increase since the 1980s) - an autoimmune disease which affects the small intestine. Symptoms include diarrhea, constipation, weight loss all which cause other health issues.

Chemotaxis - movement by a cell caused by a response to chemicals from substances that have certain chemical properties.

Chronic fatigue (11,027%) - is a state in which you are unable to do normal activities due to fatigue.

Chylomicron
Chylomicrons are lipoproteins which transport triglycerides, phospholipids, cholesterol and proteins to the adipose, cardiac and muscle cells in the body. These are formed in the small intestine. Once the material is delivered, the remnant is returned to the liver. The lipids cannot be moved through the blood on their own because lips are "oily" and the blood is watery. Oil and water don't mix.

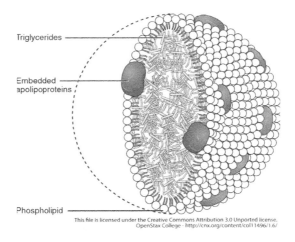

Triglycerides

Embedded apolipoproteins

Phospholipid

This file is licensed under the Creative Commons Attribution 3.0 Unported license.
OpenStax College - http://cnx.org/content/col11496/1.6/

COPD (148% increase since 1980s) - Chronic obstructive pulmonary disease. Shortness of breath because of obstructed air flow.

Coenzyme Q10 - this enzyme is critical for mitochondria (see mitochondria) to survive. Without mitochondria you would die in a few short minutes. You have about 1500 mitochondria in each of your approximately 80 trillion cells. Therefore it is estimated that you generate your body weight in ATP everyday. Statins reduce CoQ10 in the cell.

Coronary thrombosis - a narrowing of a blood vessel of the heart.

CRP - C Reactive Protein - This protein is produced by the liver in response to inflammation somewhere in the body.
See also:
High-normal levels of hs-CRP predict the development of non-alcoholic fatty liver in healthy men." - https://www.ncbi.nlm.nih.gov/pubmed/28234943

Glossary of Terms

Hyperhomocysteinemia, Insulin Resistance and High HS- CRP Levels in Prehypertension. - https://www.ncbi.nlm.nih.gov/pubmed/25302190

Type 2 diabetes mellitus and inflammation: Prospects for biomarkers of risk and nutritional intervention - https://www.ncbi.nlm.nih.gov/pmc/articles/PMC3047967/

Cytokines - regulatory proteins, such as lymphokines and interleukins that are produced by immune system cells and act as inter-cellular mediators in the modulation of immune response. - https://medical-dictionary.thefreedictionary.com/cytokines

Cytotoxic - being toxic to a cell

de novo lipogenesis - a process that converts dietary carbohydrate into fat in the time after a meal primarily in the liver but can occur in muscle and fat cells.

Diabetes (305% increase since the 1980) - high blood sugar levels over an extended period of time as a result of insulin resistance.

Dyslipidemia - an overabundant amount of fat and cholesterol found in the blood.

Eicosanoid family - Eicosanoids comprise a group of lipid mediators involved in inflammation, which include prostaglandins, thromboxanes, leukotrienes (LT) and lipoxins. - From: Studies in Natural Products Chemistry, 2016

EPOC - Excess post-exercise oxygen consumption
Excess post-exercise oxygen consumption is a measurably increased rate of oxygen intake following strenuous activity. In historical contexts the term "oxygen debt" was popularized to explain or perhaps attempt to quantify anaerobic energy expenditure, particularly as regards lactic acid/lactate metabolism; in fact, the term "oxygen debt" is still widely used to this day. Wikipedia

Etiology - the cause of a disease

Endometriosis is a condition in which bits of the tissue similar to the lining of the uterus (endometrium) grow in other parts of the body.

252

Like the uterine lining, this tissue builds up and sheds in response to monthly hormonal cycles. However, there is no natural outlet for the blood discarded from these implants. Instead, it falls onto surrounding organs, causing swelling and inflammation" - https://medical-dictionary. thefreedictionary.com/endometriosis

Endocytosis a process by which substances are brought into the cell:

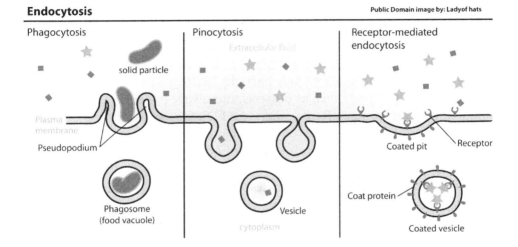

Endocytosis

Public Domain image by: Ladyof hats

Familial hypercholesterolemia - "Familial hypercholesterolemia is a disorder that is passed down through families. It causes LDL (bad) cholesterol level to be very high. The condition begins at birth and can cause heart attacks at an early age." - https://medlineplus.gov/ency/article/000392.htm

"Familial hypercholesterolemia is inherited in an autosomal dominant manner. This means that to have this condition, it is sufficient that the altered (mutated) gene is present on only one of the person's two number 19 chromosomes. A person who inherits one copy of the gene mutation causing familial hypercholesterolemia from one of his/her parents is said to have heterozygous familial hypercholesterolemia. This person has a 1 in 2 (50 percent) chance to pass on the mutated gene to each of his/her children. A person who inherits a mutated copy of the gene causing familial hypercholesterolemia from both parents is said to have homozygous familial hypercholesterolemia. This is a much more severe form of familial hypercholesterolemia than heterozygous familial hypercholesterolemia.

Each of this person's children will inherit one copy of the mutated gene and will have heterozygous familial hypercholesterolemia. " - National Human Genome Research Institute

Fats: - www.usda.gov
Saturated Fatty Acids—Fatty acids that have no double bonds. Fats high unsaturated fatty acids are usually solid-at room temperature. Major sources include animal products such as meats and dairy products, and tropical oils such as coconut.

Trans Fatty Acids—Unsaturated fatty acids that are structurally different from the unsaturated fatty acids that occur naturally in plant foods. Sources of trans fatty acids include partially hydrogenated vegetable oils used in processed foods such as desserts,microwave popcorn, frozen pizza, some margarines, and coffee creamer. (see LDL for more info.)

Ferritin - A protein that stores iron in the body.

Fibromyalgia (7,727%) - causes widespread chronic pain along with fatigue, sleep problems and problems with memory along with other issues.

GADP - Acronym for glyceraldehyde phosphate, active in metabolic pathways.

Ghrelin - is made in the gastrointestinal tract and is known as the hunger hormone. When the stomach is empty ghrelin is released and acts on the hypothalamus to stimulate hunger. Ghrelin is a part of energy homeostasis.

GIP - Gastric inhibitory polypeptide - used to stimulate insulin

GLP-1 - glaciation-like-peptide - found in the intestine the chemical slows food absorption. In the pancreas GLP-1 stimulates release of insulin. In some cases, the GLP-1 receptor in the hypothalamus reduces hunger.

Glucose - this is the source for fuel in our cells. If the cells do not get enough they will begin to die. However, too much and it becomes toxic. As levels of glucose rise, insulin is released to get the glucose into the cells. If the levels fall too much another hormone is released into the blood stream to extract glucose from the liver.

Gluconeogenesis - is the process of making glucose (for energy) from noncarbohydrate amino acids (protein) and glycerol (like triglycerides). The process takes place mainly in the liver but can also be processed in the kidneys.

Glucagon - is a hormone in the pancreas which is released to maintain glucose homeostasis. If there is not an exaggerated amount, the hormones can balance the glucose levels.

Glycolysis - "splitting sugars."

Gout occurs when the overproduction of uric acid forms tiny crystals in the joins, usually in the feet. Gout can be very painful. Usually associated with the consumption of purine-rich foods, fructose has been identified as one of the causes of gout because the toxin (uric acid) is a waste product of the liver when processing fructose.

Gynecomastia - the growth male breasts

hCG (human Chorionic Gonadotropin) - The placenta creates this hormone and is helpful in maintaining pregnancy. It causes the production of estrogen and progestrone.

Hemochromatosis - is a state where the body has too much iron in the blood. This is genetic disorder and left untreated can cause damage to the organs and joins and can be fatal.

Hematopoietic - the formation of blood cells

Hepcidin - The protein that regulates Iron in the body. Hepcidin is regulated by the HAMP gene and control the release of Iron into circulation.

Hepatic Steatosis - is the abnormal retention of fat in the liver. It can be known as Non-Alcoholic Fatty Liver Disease (NFLD)

Heterotrophs - are organisms that are cannot synthesize their own food and are thus dependent on organic sources for nutrition.

Glossary of Terms

Hyperphagia - [hahy-per-fey-jee-uh] abnormal appetite, over eating

Homosysteine - an amino acid produced when proteins are broken down.

Hyperglycemia - elevated blood sugar levels

Hypothalamus - A gland near the Pituitary gland in the brain which is responsible for the regulation of body temperature and water levels.

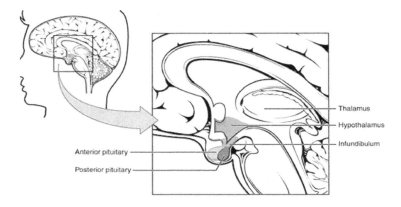

Hypothyroidism (702% increase since the 1980s) - characterized by an under active thyroid. Weight gain, feeling tired, depression intolerance for cold.

Immunotoxic - a process whereby a toxin is introduced into the cell by endocytosis and the cell is killed.

Inclusion body myositis (IBM) - a inflammatory muscle disease, an autoimmune disease that causes a slow progressive wasting of muscle tissue.

Incretins - See GLP-1

Inflammatory bowel (120% increase since the 1980s) - the inflammation of the colon and small intestine. Crohn's disease and ulcerative colitis are of this type of syndrome.

Inflammation - "inflammation of the arteries is one of the distinguishing features of atherosclerosis and coronary heart disease. In fact, chronic inflammation is associated with diabetes, obesity, Alzheimer's, cancer, and just about every other chronic degenerative disease". - Fife, Bruce.

Fat Heals, Sugar Kills: The Cause of and Cure to Cardiovascular Disease, Diabetes, Obesity, and Other Metabolic Disorders . Piccadilly Books, Ltd..

Insulin Resistance - When cells reject the chemical message from the hormone insulin and won't allow glucose to enter the cell. This will cause a host of problem unless dealt with by the diet.

In Vivo - within the living body

In Vitro - a biological process that occurs outside the body, like in a test tube.

Keytones, Ketosis - when the body creates ketone bodies out of fat and it is then used for fuel in place of sugar.

Lectins - Lectins are an "anti-nutrient" that have received much attention due to popular media and fad diet books citing lectins as a major cause for obesity, chronic inflammation, and autoimmune diseases. They are found in all plants, but raw legumes (beans, lentils, peas, soybeans, peanuts) and whole grains like wheat contain the highest amounts of lectins.
— https://www.hsph.harvard.edu/nutritionsource/anti-nutrients/lectins/

Leptin - - is made in the adipose cells and its purpose is to regulate the adipose tissue. Leptin acts on the hypothalamus in the brain to trigger that feeling of being satisfied.

LDL (low-density lipoprotein), sometimes called "bad" cholesterol. The lipoprotein is the vehicle that shuttles cholesterol around the body. There are basically two types large floating units and small dense ones. It appears that the small dense ones cause the damage when they are attacked by free radicals.

VLDL - very low-density lipoprotein

IDL - intermediate-density lipoprotein

HDL - high-density lipoprotein

LDL-C - The density of cholesterol in the lipoprotein.

LDL-P - the number of LDL particles found in the blood

oxLDL - Oxidized LDL - damaged LDL calls for macrophages and is what results in foam cells is what causes plaques and heart attacks.

sdLDL - small dense lipoproteins

Chylomicron - produced in gut to deliver ingested fats and cholesterol to the tissues

Leaky Gut Syndrome - This is an instance where the lining of the intestine is compromised, junctions between cells are loosen allowing antigens (a molecule that activates a immune response) to exit the intestine and enter the blood stream. This is thought to cause celiac disease and other autoimmune diseases. Leaky gut allows glutamate to enter the blood stream. Glutamate is a neurotoxin which causes cellular death in the brain and nervous system.

Lipogenesis - is the conversion of carbohydrates into fat for storage. This is then assumability will be used for fuel in the future. It forms triglycerides, these are put into very low-density lipoproteins (VLDL) and sent into circulation where the adipose (fat cells) stores it.

Lipoproteins - a structure used to transport cholesterol through the blood and the Extracellular fluid (ECF) fluid outside the cell. Cholesterol is a type of fat and cannot move through the blood without a transport.

Lysosomes - from the Greek words lysis "to loosen", and soma, "body". It is referred to as the ,"stomach" of the cell. It is a vesicle with the function of digesting bacteria and waste. It contains a wide variety of enzymes to accomplish its task. Some refer to it as, "suicide sacs" because it will merge with phagosomes to self-digest the cell effectively killing it.

Metabolic Syndrome - is the combination of five disorders which are usually found together: High fasting glucose, Abdominal obesity, high amount of triglycerides, low HDL cholesterol and high blood pressure. These will eventually, if not dealt with appropriately, lead to diabetes, heart disease, Alzheimer along with other issues. Some issues will cascade into other deadly illnesses. The major contributing factor is insulin resistance.

Mitochondria - The mitochondria is an organelle found in eukaryotic (cells with a nucleus) cells that perform cellular respiration among other things. Cellular respiration is a series of chemical reactions through which glucose is converted into the energy carrier - ATP. The mitochondria have its own genome (mtDNA). This is separate and distinct from the DNA found in the nucleus. This mtDNA originates only from your mother. There is more going on in the mitochondria, but we will focus on the ATP synthase. ATP is generated by converting the ADP molecule, (adenosine diphosphate) by adding a third phosphate unit. The ATP synthase has a wheel-like structure that turns up to 200 times per second and produces three ATP molecules on each turn, resulting in six hundred new ATPs per second. Each cell is estimated to have about one billion ATP molecules at any one time. However, this is only enough to last a few minutes and ADP is recycled to ATP continuously.

You need ATP to move your muscles among many other things. ATP is not stable enough to be sent to the muscle through the blood so it must be available at the cell level. It is incredible that there are many of these molecular machines manufacturing ATP 24/7. It takes ATP to make ATP so the question we need to ask the evolutionist is: "How did life exist before ATP?"

> "The supply of ATP must be steady because its lack would kill an organism in a matter of minutes. Poisons like cyanide kill so quickly by blocking processing of ATP according to Bergman". *ATP: The Perfect Energy Currency for the Cell by* Jerry Bergman, CRSQ Vol 36(1) June, 1999.

Mitochondrial DNA - is DNA found in the mitochondria. It is typically inherited from the mother. Mitochondrial DNA is a circular closed double helix with approximately 17,000 base pares as compared to DNA in the cell which has three billion.

Dr. Bryan Sykes wrote a book called The Seven Daughters of Eve. Dr. Sykes investigated the mtDNA found in a 5000 year old frozen Italian. He found that the DNA was the same as that in modern Europeans. In one case, he found that the mtDNA was the same, making them and the others genetically linked.

Glossary of Terms

The title of Sykes book comes from the fact that 95% of Europe's population comes from just seven haplogroups. Haplogroups define differences in human mitochondrial DNA. Sykes identified them by the letters U, X, H, V, T, K, and J and further gave them names; Ursula, Xenia, Helena, Velda, Tara, Katrine, and Jasmine. The Europeans could now trace their lineage back to a common mother.

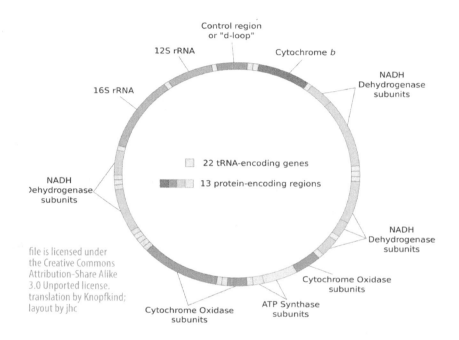

Multiple sclerosis (117%) - A disease of the nerve cells. The myelin sheath, which are insulating covers on the nervous system is damaged. Myelin is 40% water the rest is made up of 60-75% lipid (fat) and 15-25% protein.

Myocardial Infarction - heart attack

Myositis - the term myositis is used to refer to a disease involving chronic inflammation of the muscles, often occurring together with other symptoms. This condition is also known as idiopathic inflammatory myopathy (IIM). The disease is highly variable and has been classified into a number of forms, including dermatomyositis (DM), polymyositis (PM), necrotizing myopathy (NM), sporadic inclusion body myositis (sIBM), and juvenile forms of myositis (JM). - The Myositis Association - www.myositis.org/

Microbiome - Microorganisms living in the body mostly in the digestive track. "The human microbiota consists of the 10–100 trillion symbiotic microbial cells harbored by each person, primarily bacteria in the gut." - Department of Chemistry & Biochemistry at the University of Colorado

Neurotoxic - the harmful effects to the nervous system by a biological, or chemical substance.

Neurotrophins - chemicals that support neuron function and synapse formation for enhanced cognitive function.

Obesogens may be functionally defined as chemicals that inappropriately alter lipid homeostasis and fat storage, change metabolic set points, disrupt energy balance or modify the regulation of appetite and satiety to promote fat accumulation and obesity. - Kirchner S, Kieu T, Chow C, Casey S, Blumberg B (March 2010). *"Prenatal exposure to the environmental obesogen tributyltin predisposes multipotent stem cells to become adipocytes"*

Osteoarthritis (449% increase since the 1980s) -

Polycystic ovary syndrome - this is the result of elevated male hormones in females. Generally speaking you will find excess body hair, heavy menstrual periods, mood disorders and infertility.

Polysaccharide - A polysaccharide is a large molecule made of many smaller monosaccharides. Monosaccharides are simple sugars, like glucose. - *Biology Dictionary*

PUFA - Polyunsaturated fats a cause of oxidative stress in the body.

Prostaglandin member of the eicosanoid - Biochemistry. any of a class of unsaturated fatty acids that are involved in the contraction of smooth muscle, the control of inflammation and body temperature, and many other physiological functions. - www.dictionary.com

ROS - (Reactive oxygen species) A type of unstable molecule that contains oxygen and that easily reacts with other molecules in a cell. A build up of reactive oxygen species in cells may cause damage to DNA, RNA, and proteins, and may cause cell death. Reactive oxygen species are free radicals. Also called oxygen radical. — National Cancer Institute Dictionary of Cancer Terms

Ruminant - Ruminants are mammals that are able to acquire nutrients from plant-based food by fermenting it in a specialized stomach prior to digestion, principally through microbial actions - Wikipedia, The Free Encyclopedia, 6 Aug. 2019. Web. 8 Aug. 2019.

Sleep apnea (430% increase since the 1980s) - pauses in breathing during sleep, snoring and sleepy during the day.

Statins - This is a drug that brings in billions of dollars to the drug manufactures, Pfizerís statin drug Lipitor, had $10.9 billion in sales in a single year, 2004 - Pfizer. 2004 Financial Report. Available at: www.pfizer.com/pfizer/annualreport/2004/financial/financial2004.pdf. Its stated purpose is to lower LDL cholesterol, the so called "bad cholesterol". However, in recent studies the effectiveness of such drugs have not proven to help all that much in patients.

According to David Diamond and Dr. Ravnskov, statins produce a dramatic reduction in cholesterol levels, but they have "failed to substantially improve cardiovascular outcomes." They further state that the many studies touting the efficacy of statins have not only neglected to account for the numerous serious adverse side effects of the drugs, but supporters of statins have used what the authors refer to as "statistical deception" to make inflated claims about their effectiveness.

— *Efficacy of Statins Exaggerated* - Author: University of South Florida (USF Health)(i) : Contact: Adam Freeman/David Diamond - ddiamond@usf.edu Published: 2015-02-20 : (Rev. 2019-11-21)

Appendix
C

Medical Doctors
And
Other Resources

*This **is not** an exhaustive list, but some resources I have learned from during my journey to good health. I think you will benefit from these resources*

Alphabetically (This is a short list of Doctors, Scientists, books and websites)

Christian Assad-Kottner, MD

Description from Ketomojo

Dr. Assad-Kottner is an Interventional Cardiologist who has a deep interest in the application of Lifestyle Medicine to prevent and reverse disease. He is the Director of The CardioMetabolic Clinic in RGV Cardiology, McAllen Texas. In addition to his passion for Lifestyle, he has a deep interest in the incorporation of technology to improve healthcare. He was one of the first MDs to utilize augmented and virtual reality in the healthcare setting. He and his team were the first to show proof of concept of Tele-Mentoring procedures via augmented Reality Glasses (Google Glass).

Dr. Assad-Kottner is also a pioneer in the incorporation of Virtual Reality in the Healthcare setting making his own recordings and videos with personally modified equipment at the time which later led him to work with JauntVR and experiment with proof of concept of Virtual Reality in Medical Education. Dr. Assad-Kottner also has award winning research done in The Methodist DeBakey Heart Center regarding Heart Failure where he discovered a strong presence of Anti-Cardiac Antibodies in the failing myocardium. He is a former faculty of Singularity University where he became a Co-Founder of a TeleHealth platform aiming to democratize healthcare around the world. Since he started his practice in McAllen Texas, recently named the most obese city in the United States, Dr. Assad-Kottner became frustrated in regards to the health issues affecting a majority of the population at his current city; for this reason, he decided to modify his approach in care from Intervention to Prevention. Instead of focusing on sick-care he actively focuses on Health-Care aiming to prevent the catastrophic complications of Obesity, Diabetes, and Cardiovascular disease.

Website: https://www.doximity.com/pub/christian-assad-kottner-md

---

Dr. Peter Attia M.D.

Peter is the founder of Attia Medical, PC, a medical practice with offices in San Diego and New York City, focusing on the applied science of longevity. The practice applies nutritional biochemistry, exercise physiology, sleep physiology, techniques to increase distress tolerance, lipidology, pharmacology, and four-system endocrinology to increase lifespan (delaying the onset of chronic disease), while simultaneously improving health span (quality of life).

Website: https://peterattiamd.com/

Dr. Nadir Ali M.D.

Dr. Nadir Ali is an interventional cardiologist with over 25 years of experience. He is also the chairman of the Department of Cardiology at Clear Lake Regional Medical Center. Before working as a cardiologist, he served as an assistant professor of medicine for eight years at Baylor College of Medicine in Houston, where he also received his medical training.

Dr. Ali has championed many aspects of the science and practice of a low-carb lifestyle in the local Clear Lake area since 2013. He organizes a monthly nutritional seminar in the Searcy Auditorium of the Clear Lake Hospital that receives more than 100 visitors every month from the local community. Dr Ali's focus is on managing heart disease, obesity, metabolic syndrome and diabetes

---

Dr. Shawn Baker

Dr. Shawn Baker completed his undergraduate degree at the University of Texas in Austin. He graduated with honors from Texas Tech Medical School and completed his Internship and Orthopedic Surgery Residency at the University of Texas Medical Branch in Galveston.

He is a lifelong multi-sport elite-level athlete who served as a combat trauma surgeon and chief of orthopedics while deployed to Afghanistan with the United States Air Force. His lifelong passion for athletics and strength training has resulted in numerous state and national weightlifting records and a semi- professional rugby career. His focus in recent years has been on using nutrition as a tool for health, performance, and overall well-being.

Book:	The Carnivore Diet
Website:	https://www.shawn-baker.com/

Dr. James R. Bailes - M.D.

Dr. Bailes is a pediatric endocrinologist and co-author of *No More Fat Kids, a Pediatrician's Guide for Safe and Effective Weight Loss.*
He specializes in childhood obesity and is also an Associate Professor of Pediatrics at Marshall University, School of Medicine, in Huntington, WV.
Dr. Bailes has developed a health program for school-age children, allowing them to lose weight without feeling hungry. His straightforward, practical and easy to follow approach is said to improve overall health, lipid profiles and most importantly, self-esteem.

Book:	No More Fat Kids: A Pediatrician's Guide For Safe & Effective Weight Loss - Avant Garde Publishing

---

Dr. Ken Berry M.D.

Dr. Ken Berry is a family medicine doctor in Camden, Tennessee and is affiliated with Henry County Medical Center. He received his medical degree from University of Tennessee College of Medicine and has been in practice between 11-20 years. He is one of 11 doctors at Henry County Medical Center who specialize in Family Medicine.

Website:	https://www.kendberrymd.com/
Book:	Lies My Doctor Told Me

Dr. Benjamin Bikman Ph.D.

His Ph.D. in Bioenergetics and was a postdoctoral fellow with the Duke-National University of Singapore in metabolic disorders. He is currently a professor of pathophysiology and a biomedical scientist at Brigham Young University in Utah.

268

Website: https://bikmanlab.byu.edu/

Dr. David Brownstein M.D.

Dr. David Brownstein is a Board-Certified family physician and is one of the foremost practitioners of holistic medicine. He is the Medical Director of the Center for Holistic Medicine in West Bloomfield, MI.

Books: Heal Your Leaky Gut: The Hidden Cause of Many Chronic Diseases
Overcoming Thyroid Disorders
Iodine : Why You Need It, Why You Can't Live Without It

Website: https://www.drbrownstein.com/about-drbrownstein/

Peter Brukner, MD, OAM, MBBS, FACSP, FACSM, FASMF, FFSEM
(description from https://lowcarbconferences.com/peter-brukner-md/)

Dr Brukner has had two passions during this medical career.
The first was sports medicine. Peter is a world renowned sports medicine clinician and researcher. He was the founding partner at the Olympic Park Sports Medicine Centre in Melbourne, has served two terms as president of the Australasian College of Sports Physicians, is the co-author of the 'bible' of sports medicine Brukner & Khan's Clinical Sports Medicine, and has been team doctor to amateur and professional sporting teams such as Melbourne and Collingwood (AFL), National swimming, hockey, athletics, soccer and cricket teams as well as Liverpool Football Club in the English Premier league. Peter is Professor of Sports Medicine at La Trobe University in Melbourne.

Website: https://www.peterbrukner.com/
Books: A Fat Lot of Good: How the Experts Got Food and Diet So
Wrong and What You Can Do to Take Back Control of
Your Health

Dr. Duane Graveline MD - (deceased - 2016)

Duane Graveline M.D., M.P.H. earned his Doctor of Medicine degree from the University of Vermont College of Medicine in June 1955. He then spent a year as an intern at Walter Reed Army Hospital followed by a year as Chief of Aviation Medicine Service at Kelly Air Force Base. In 1958 Dr. Graveline received a Master's degree in Public Health from Johns Hopkins School of Hygiene and Public Health. An Aerospace Medical residency followed at the Air Force School of Aerospace Medicine and he completed residency training at Brooks Air Force Base receiving specialty certification by the American Board in Preventative Medicine. In 1962 Dr. Graveline was designated a NASA flight controller for the Mercury and Gemini program.

Books: The Dark Side of Statins: Plus: The Wonder of Cholesterol
Lipitor® Thief of Memory
Statin Drugs Side Effects and the Misguided War on Cholesterol
The Statin Damage Crisis

Website: https://spacedoc.com/

Dr. David Cavan MD

Dr David Cavan is one of the UK's leading experts on diabetes self-management. He worked for many years as a Consultant at the highly-regarded Bournemouth Diabetes and Endocrine Centre. He is now the Director of Policy and Programs at the International Diabetes Federation, whose mission is to promote diabetes care, prevention and a cure worldwide. www.diabetes.co.uk is the UK's largest and fastest-growing community website and forum for people with diabetes.

Books: Reverse Your Diabetes: The Step-by-Step Plan to Take Control of Type 2 Diabetes

Website: https://www.drdavidcavan.com/

DR. DOMINIC D`AGOSTINO

Website   https://www.ketonutrition.org/

Books: Tripping over the Truth: How the Metabolic Theory of Cancer Is Overturning One of Medicine's Most Entrenched Paradigms - by Travis Christofferson (Dr. D'Agostino wrote forward to the book)

William Davis MD

Dr. William Davis is responsible for exposing the incredible nutritional blunder being made by "official" health agencies: Eat more "healthy whole grains." The wheat of today is different from the wheat of 1960, thanks to extensive genetics manipulations introduced to increase yield-per-acre. Founder of the international on-line program for heart health, Track Your Plaque, his experience in thousands of participants uncovered how foods made of wheat actually CAUSED heart disease and heart attack. Eliminating wheat yielded results beyond everyone's expectations: substantial weight loss, correction of cholesterol abnormalities, relief from inflammatory diseases like arthritis, better mood--benefits that led to prevention of heart disease but a lot more benefits in other areas of health.

Dr. Davis now advocates a lifestyle in which all foods made from wheat are removed. He articulates this approach in his book, Wheat Belly: Lose the wheat, lose the weight and find your path back to health, as well as his on-line program, Track Your Plaque (www.trackyourplaque.com). He lives what he preaches, not having indulged in a wheat-containing bagel, ciabatta, or pretzel in many years. Dr. Davis practices preventive cardiology in Milwaukee, Wisconsin. (description fromAmazon.com)

Books: Undoctored: Why Health Care Has Failed You and How You Can Become Smarter Than Your Doctor

Wheat Belly: Lose the Wheat, Lose the Weight, and Find Your Path Back to Health

Website: https://www.wheatbellyblog.com/

Dr. Georgia Ede, Psychiatric

I first became interested in nutrition after discovering a new way of eating that completely reversed a number of perplexing health problems I had developed in my early 40s, including Chronic Fatigue Syndrome, Fibromyalgia, Migraines, and IBS. This experience led me on a quest to understand why the unorthodox diet that restored my own health is so different from the diet we are taught is healthy. (from her website)

Website: https://www.diagnosisdiet.com

Dr. Andreas Enfelt, M.D.

The Doctor received his Ph.D. in Biology in 1985, with a specialization in Behavioral Neuroscientist, from the Center for the Neurobiology of Learning and Memory at the University of California, Irvine. Dr. Eenfeldt spent twelve years working as a doctor and eight of those years as a family physician, treating patients with low-carb, high-fat diets. During that time he witnessed amazing success for people with obesity and type 2 diabetes.

Website: https://www.dietdoctor.com

Dr. Gary Fettke

Dr. Gary Fettke, an orthopedic surgeon from Tasmania. A brain cancer survivor, he has lectured around the world about the importance of nutrition in chronic diseases such as cancer. I met him in Cape Town, South Africa where he impressed me, not so much with his boyish good looks (alright, not very much at all for this) but his deep understanding and passion for nutrition. As fellow doctors, I fully understand the critical importance of nutrition in metabolic disease. (from dietdoctor.com)

Like Dr. Noakes he was censured by the Dietetic Association and told not to recommend a low sugar, low carbohydrate diet to his patients any longer. Dr. Fettke was eventually cleared and can now recommend the diet changes.

Website: http://www.nofructose.com

Dr. Jason Fung, Nephrologist

Dr. Jason Fung is a Canadian nephrologist (specialty of medicine and pediatrics that concerns itself with the kidneys:). He's a world-leading expert on intermittent fasting and low carb, especially for treating people with type 2 diabetes. He has written three best-selling health books and he co-founded the Intensive Dietary Management program.

Books: The Obesity Code: Unlocking the Secrets of Weight Loss
    The Longevity Solution: Rediscovering Centuries-Old
    Secrets to a Healthy, Long Life

Dr. Jeffry Gerber MD

He offers a full range of family medicine services including primary care, preventive medicine, acute and episodic care, Nutrition Counseling & Medical Weight Loss. Most of ones' health care needs can be addressed at our office. Since 1993 we have developed a network with many specialists here in the Denver metro area to ensure complete and comprehensive care for the individual or family.

Books: Eat Rich, Live Long: Mastering the Low-Carb & Keto
          Spectrum for Weight Loss and Longevity
Website: https://jgerbermd.com/

Dr. Joesph Kraft M.D.

A medical doctor who measured 14,384 people ages 3 to 90 with his oral glucose tolerance tests. This is a standard test to measure the blood glucose response to a standardized amount of glucose over 2 hours. The difference is that he measured over 5 hours and included blood insulin levels. Out of all those tested only 25% had normal blood glucose and were not diabetic.

Books: Diabetes Epidemic and You - Trafford Publishing

Dr. Malcom Kendrick, GP

Malcolm graduated in medicine and now lives and works in sunny Cheshire as a General Practitioner. He has always tried to question received wisdom where it seems flawed which, to him, seems to be all over the place. He wrote The Great Cholesterol Con as it became clear that the accepted ideas on diet, Cholesterol and heart disease were bunk. He has his own blog drmalcolmkendrick.org where he discusses a wide range of health issues.

He tries to live according to his own philosophy on health which is simple. Enjoy life, enjoy friends and family, do a bit of exercise, and don't worry too much.

Books: Doctoring Data

The Great Cholesterol Con

Website: https://drmalcolmkendrick.org/

Dr. Chris Knobbe - Description from Low Carb Denver 2020

Dr. Chris Knobbe is an ophthalmologist and Associate Clinical Professor Emeritus, formerly of the University of Texas Southwestern Medical Center, in Dallas, Texas. He is also the founder and president of Cure AMD Foundation, a nonprofit organisation dedicated to the prevention of vision loss from age-related macular degeneration (AMD).

Dr. Knobbe has a deep interest in general nutrition, particularly as it relates to chronic degenerative disease, though his primary area of expertise is with the disorder AMD. AMD is the leading cause of irreversible vision loss and blindness in people over the age of 65, currently affecting approximately 196 million people worldwide.

Books: Ancestral Dietary Strategy to Prevent and Treat Macular Degeneration.

Website: https://www.cureamd.org

Michael Garrett, MD

A family medicine doctor in Austin, Texas and is affiliated with Hospital at Westlake Medical Center. He received his M.D. from Indiana University School of Medicine in 1997, and completed residency in Family Medicine at Ball Memorial Hospital in 2000. After 14 years of Emergency Medicine, he opened Direct MD Austin, a full service direct primary care practice. He is a founding member of the DPC Alliance, and has been using low-carb and ketogentic diets for years to reverse metabolic diseases and optimize health

---

Dr. Sarah Hallberg, M.D.

Dr. Sarah Hallberg, DO is an internal medicine specialist in Lafayette, IN and has been practicing for 17 years. She graduated from Des Moines University, College Of Osteopathic Medicine and Surgery in 2002 and specializes in internal medicine

Dr. Sarah Hallberg is the Medical Director at Virta Health, the first clinically-proven treatment to safely and sustainability reverse type 2 diabetes without medications or surgery.

Website: https://www.virtahealth.com/about/drsarahhallberg

Dr. Christy Kesslering MD

Dr. Kesslering is passionate about how diet and lifestyle impact cancer incidence and recurrence rates and works with patients to make positive changes.

When asked why she chose Radiation Oncology, she states, "I love being able to teach my patients about their disease and to help in their cure or to alleviate their symptoms and improve their quality of life. I also enjoy the constantly changing technical side of radiation oncology."

Website:
https://www.chicagocancer.org/meet-our-team/christy-m-kesslering-md

---

Dr. Dwight Lundell, M.D.

Dr. Dwight Lundell received training in Cardiovascular and Thoracic surgery from Yale University and have performed over 5,000 open heart surgeries. Inducted into The Beating Heart Hall of Fame.

During his successful career, He had a unique vantage point peering into thousands of hearts and arteries. And what he saw was shocking. Cholesterol lowering drugs and many others for diabetes and blood pressure weren't helping my beloved patients.

He watched as countless heart attack victims lost their health to the misguided war on cholesterol and the use of prescription drugs. When he spoke out, he was scorned and labeled a quack.

Regardless, he continued "confessing" what he had viewed under the lights of the sterile operating room. And he guided his patients toward better lifestyle habits and botanical medicine. Thousands began reversing decades of poor health, naturally.

Threatening his hospital's revenue stream, the medical license that he was no longer using was officially revoked. Confessions of a Maverick Heart

Surgeon (And Iron-man) are the stories they don't want public...and the ones that can help you make a true health comeback!

Website: https://www.drlundellmd.com
Book:

Brian Lenzkes, MD

Dr. Lenzkes is a USC trained, board certified Internal Medicine doctor and has been in practice for 16 years but did not understand the implications of metabolic syndrome until only a few years ago. He has had a personal struggle with obesity since childhood and became officially pre-diabetic in February of 2017 despite his medical knowledge. Although Dr. Lenzkes was voted one of the "Top Doctors" in San Diego for 11 of those years, he still felt a void as many of my patients with chronic conditions continued to decline and require more medication. After attending LowCarbUSA ® in San Diego, his practice of medicine changed and he have taken control of his health. Dr. Lenzkes has been honored to be a guest on multiple podcasts and I has been a speaker on the Nutrition Network educational series for medical professionals. He is currently co-hosting the Low Carb MD podcast with Dr. Jason Fung, Dr. Tro Kalayjian, and Megan Ramos. He is also on the panel of advisers for the LowCarbUSA ® Clinical Guidelines for Medical Professionals and recorded an interview for the documentary; Big Fat Lie with Wide Eye Productions. Brian is the CEO of Low Carb MD San Diego. He believes that together we can do our part to reverse the healthcare crisis that is facing the world one life at a time. Dr. Lenzkes is excited about the journey ahead.

Robert H. Lustig, M.D.

American pediatric endocrinologist. He is Professor of Pediatrics in the Division of Endocrinology at the University of California, San Francisco, where he specializes in neuroendocrinology and childhood obesity. He is also director of UCSF's WATCH program, and president and co-founder of the non-profit Institute for Responsible Nutrition. - Wikipedia

Books: Fat Chance
                 The Hacking of the American Mind: The Science Behind
                       the Corporate Takeover of Our Bodies and Brains

Website: https://robertlustig.com/

Dr. Aseem Malhotra, M.D.

Award-winning cardiologist, Dr Aseem Malhotra, is successfully leading the campaign against excess sugar consumption and calls for greater transparency in patient care. Known as one of the most influential cardiologists in Britain, Dr Aseem Malhotra is successfully leading the campaign against excess sugar consumption.

Books: The Pioppi Diet: A 21-Day Lifestyle Plan.

Website: https://doctoraseem.com/

Dr Paul Mason

He obtained his medical degree with honors from the University of Sydney, and also holds degrees in Physiotherapy and Occupational Health. He is a Specialist Sports Medicine and Exercise Physician. Dr Mason also has an in depth understanding of the latest science surrounding weight loss and nutrition. Using a low carbohydrate approach, he helps his patients achieve excellent results

---

Dr. Natasha Campbell-McBride

Dr. Natasha Campbell-McBride is a warm, gracious woman with a revolutionary mission — helping people to heal their minds and bodies and avoid a wide array of disorders and illnesses by focusing on supporting gut health. The experience of having a child with autism propelled her to look beyond the confines of conventional medicine and to become a medical pioneer. She is best known for the GAPS Nutritional Protocol. GAPS is the acronym for both Gut and Psychology Syndrome and Gut and Physiology Syndrome. Campbell-McBride graduated with Honors as a medical doctor in Russia in 1984 and later received a graduate degree in Neurology. After working as a neurologist and a neurosurgeon for a total of eight years, she started a family and moved to England. During that time she developed her theories on the relationship between neurological disorders and nutrition, and completed a second graduate degree in Human Nutrition at Sheffield University, UK. In 2000 she started the Cambridge Nutrition Clinic, where she specializes in nutritional approaches to treat learning disabilities and other psychological disorders, as well as digestive and immune disorders, in both children and adults. (description from: Eco Farming Daily)

Book: Gut and Psychology Syndrome: Natural Treatment for Autism, Dyspraxia, A.D.D., Dyslexia, A.D.H.D., Depression, Schizophrenia

---

Dr. Dariush Mozaffarian, DrPh, MPH, MD, BS

(description from denverdietdoctor.com)
Jean Mayer Professor of Nutrition and Medicine, and Dean of the Friedman School of Nutrition Science & Policy, Tufts University. Dariush Mozaffarian is Dean of the Tufts Friedman School of Nutrition Science & Policy, and the Jean Mayer Chair and Professor of Nutrition. The only graduate school of nutrition in North America, the Friedman School produces trusted science and real-world impact in nutrition. A board-certified cardiologist and epidemiologist, Dr. Mozaffarian's research focuses on how diet and lifestyle influence cardiometabolic health and how effective policies can reduce these burdens. He has authored nearly 300 scientific publications on dietary fats, foods, and diet patterns; global obesity, diabetes, and cardiovascular diseases; and evidence-based and cost-effective dietary policies. Dr. Mozaffarian has served in numerous advisory roles including for the US and Canadian governments, American

Heart Association, Global Burden of Diseases study, World Health Organization, and United Nations. His work has been featured in the New York Times, Washington Post, Wall Street Journal, National Public Radio, Time Magazine, and countless other news outlets, broadcasts, blogs, and websites.

Dr. Mozaffarian received his BS in biological sciences from Stanford (Phi Beta Kappa), MD from Columbia (Alpha Omega Alpha), and trained in internal medicine and cardiovascular medicine at Stanford and U. of Washington. Following his clinical training, he received his MPH from U. of Washington and Doctorate in Public Health from Harvard. Before he was appointed Dean at Tufts in 2014, Dr. Mozaffarian was on the faculty at Harvard Medical School and Harvard School of Public Health for a decade and was clinically active on the cardiology service at Brigham and Women's Hospital. He is married with three children and a second degree Black Belt in Tae Kwon Do.

Dr. Adam Nally D.O.

Adam S. Nally, D.O., (popularly known as @DocMuscles), is the go-to no-nonsense community-based physician providing practical weight management & general medical health through a distinctly individualized ketogentic, low-carbohydrate, and/or paleolithic lifestyle combined with a cutting edge medical approach. With over twenty years of practical, in-the-trenches, medical experience and an enchantingly passionate, articulate, & genuine approach to the treatment of the "diseases of civilization," you're going to want him on your medical team.

Book: The Keto Cure: A Low Carb High Fat Dietary Solution to Heal Your Body and Optimize Your Health

Website: https://www.patreon.com/docmuscles

Professor Tim Noakes M.D.

Timothy David Noakes is a South African scientist, and an emeritus professor in the Division of Exercise Science and Sports Medicine at the

University of Cape Town. He is also a member of the National Research Foundation of South Africa, who list him as one of their highest-rated members.- Wikipedia

Tim was Dragged in to court by an incensed dietitian because of a tweet suggesting a low carb diet.

Books: Lore of Nutrition - Challenging Conventional Dietary
Beliefs
The Real Meal Revolution: The Radical, Sustainable
Approach to Healthy Eating
Real Food On Trial: How the diet dictators tried to destroy
a top scientist
Diabetes Unpacked: Just Science and Sense. No Sugar
Coating

Website: www.Thenoakesfoundation.org

Dr. Tim O'Dowd

Born and educated in Ireland, Dr. Tim O'Dowd arrived in Australia as a newly qualified doctor in 1975. He initially trained in obstetric and gynecology at the Mater Hospital in Brisbane and gained specialist qualifications in England (FRCOG) and Australia (FRANZCOG).

Dr Stephen Phinney, MD, PhD,

Stephen Phinney is the Chief Medical Officer and Co-Founder of Virta Health, the first clinically-proven treatment to safely and sustainability reverse type 2 diabetes without medications or surgery. As a physician-scientist with 40 years of experience divided between academic internal medicine and industry, Dr. Phinney has studied nutritional biochemistry with a long-term focus on low carbohydrate research and its benefits for physical performance and insulin sensitivity. His career has emphasized the interaction between diet and exercise and their effects on obesity, body composition, physical performance, and cellular membrane structure

Book: The Art and Science of Low Carbohydrate Performance

Website: https://www.virtahealth.com/about/drstephenphinney

Dr. Luan Pho MD

is board-certified in internal medicine and is also a wound care specialist. He has been in private practice for over a decade. After receiving an undergraduate degree in Biology from Southern Methodist University, he earned his medical degree at the University of Texas Medical Center Houston, and completed his residency at the Presbyterian Hospital of Dallas. He, his wife, and their three girls live in the suburb of Dallas, Texas.

Book: Health and Vitality Truths

Website: http://www.luanphomd.com/

Dr. Paul Saladino

Dr. Saladino is the leading authority on the science and application of the carnivore diet. He has used this diet to reverse autoimmunity, chronic inflammation and mental health issues in hundreds of patients, many of whom had been told their conditions were untreatable.

Book: The Carnivore Code: Unlocking the Secrets to Optimal Health by Returning to Our Ancestral Diet

Website: https://carnivoremd.com/

Dr. Uffe Ravnskov

Uffe Ravnskov is a Danish medical doctor, independent researcher, a member of various international scientific organizations, and a former assistant professor and medical practitioner in Denmark and Sweden. In recent years he has gained notoriety for questioning the scientific consensus regarding the Lipid Hypothesis - Wikipedia

Book: The Cholestrol Myth

Website: http://www.ravnskov.nu/cholesterol/

Dr. Stephanie Seneff, Ph.D.,

Senior Research Scientist at the MIT Computer Science and Artificial Intelligence Laboratory. Dr. Seneff holds multiple degrees from MIT including: Undergraduate Degree in Biophysics, M.S. and E.E. in Electrical Engineering, and Ph. D in Electrical Engineering and Computer Science. Research Focus: Compilation & Analysis of Epidemiological Data to Determine Risk Factors for Illness & Disease.

Book: Cindy & Erica's Obsession to Solve Today's Health Care Crisis: Autism, Alzheimer's Disease, Cardiovascular Disease, ALS and More

Website: https://people.csail.mit.edu/seneff/

Dr. Cate Shanahan MD

Dr. Shanahan is a board certified Family Physician. After getting her BS in biology from Rutgers University, she trained in biochemistry and genetics at Cornell University's graduate school before attending Robert Wood Johnson Medical School. She practiced in Hawaii for ten years where she studied ethnobotany and her healthiest patient's culinary habits. She applied her learning and experiences in all these scientific fields to write Deep Nutrition: Why Your Genes Need Traditional Food. Together with Dr. Tim DiFrancesco and NBA legend Gary Vitti, she created the PRO Nutrition program for the LA Lakers. In May of 2019 she will begin consulting work as Director of Metabolic Health for ABC Fine Wine and Spirits, a progressive, family run company interested in saving money by betterment of health. She also consults for athletic teams in the NYC area and remotely. - Quote from her website

Books: Deep Nutrition

Website: www.drcate.com

Dr. Bret Scher

As the low Carb Cardiologist and medical director at DietDoctor.com, I want to help you achieve extraordinary health and happiness. By using a healthy low carb lifestyle, you can transform your health and your life. Let's face it. Our healthcare system is broken and leaves us confused, unclear how to achieve our health goals. You can break free and live exceptionally! Explore my website, follow my blog, listen to my podcasts, and let me know how I can help you on your journey to Your Best Health Ever! Thanks for making your health a priority!

Website: http://www.drbretscher.com/
https://dietdoctor.com

Book: Your Best Health Ever!: The Cardiologist's Surprisingly Simple Guide to What Really Works

---

Dr. Roy Taylor

"Roy Taylor qualified in medicine at the University of Edinburgh, and is Professor of Medicine and Metabolism at Newcastle University and Newcastle Hospitals NHS Trust. He has been conducting research on type 2 diabetes since 1978[4]. He founded the Newcastle Magnetic Resonance Centre in 2006 to apply innovative techniques to study in all medical specialties.

In 2011 he showed that type 2 diabetes was a simple, reversible condition of excess fat within liver and pancreas. This led to a series of studies, most recently the Diabetes Remission Clinical Trial which demonstrated that type 2 diabetes can be reversed to normal in Primary Care and that the underlying pathophysiological changes were durable.

Professor Taylor developed the system now used through the United Kingdom for screening for diabetic eye disease, with major reduction in blindness due to diabetes across the UK. He has produced books and other teaching aids for retinal screeners and co-founded the British Association of Retinal Screeners. He developed the Newcastle Obstetric Medical service and advanced clinical management in diabetes and in hyperemesis."

From: Wikipedia contributors, "Roy Taylor (scientist)," Wikipedia, The Free Encyclopedia, https://en.wikipedia.org/w/index.php?title=Roy_Taylor_(scientist)&oldid=951375334 (accessed June 10, 2020).

Books: Life Without Diabetes: The definitive guide to understanding and reversing your type 2 diabetes

---

Dr. Simon Thornley

Dr Simon Thornley is an epidemiologist, lecturer, researcher and Public Health Physician working at the University of Auckland in the section of Epidemiology and Biostatistics. After training in medicine, Simon worked as a junior doctor in all three large hospitals in the Auckland region, as well as in the Hunter Valley region in New South Wales, Australia.

Since then, Dr. Thornley retrained in public health medicine and has been working in academia and the health sector in epidemiological and public health roles. His research interests include tobacco dependence, food addiction and obesity, cardiovascular disease, diabetes, psychiatric disease, injury and environmental epidemiology. He has an interest in the health effects of sugar and low carb lifestyles

---

Dr. David Unwin, MD

Dr. Unwin is known for pioneering the low-carb approach in his profession in the UK. In 2016 he won the prestigious NHS Innovator of the Year award for his work with diabetes patients. On top of that, Dr. Unwin is the medical advisor at the popular Low Carb Program and is doing his best to spread knowledge about low carb among doctors, dietitians and nurses.

(description from dietdoctor.com)

Dr. Eric Westman, MD

Dr. Westman is also director of the Duke University Lifestyle Medicine Clinic which he founded in 2006 after conducting many scientific studies on the advantage of keto lifestyle and diet – and after converting his own medical practice to the treatment of diabetes, obesity and other diseases with a ketogentic approach

Book: Keto Clarity: Your Definitive Guide to the Benefits of a Low-Carb, High-Fat Diet
The New Atkins for a New You: The Ultimate Diet for Shedding Weight and Feeling Great

Website: https://www.dukehealth.org/find-doctors-physicians /eric-c-westman-md-mhs

Dr. Terry Wahls, MD

Description from her website:
Dr. Terry Wahls is a clinical professor of medicine at the University of Iowa where she conducts clinical trials. She is also a patient with secondary progressive multiple sclerosis, which confined her to a tilt-recline wheelchair for four years. Dr. Wahls restored her health using a diet and lifestyle program she designed specifically for her brain and now pedals her bike to work each day. She is the author of The Wahls Protocol: How I Beat Progressive MS Using Paleo Principles and Functional Medicine, The Wahls Protocol: A Radical New Way to Treat All Chronic Autoimmune Conditions Using Paleo Principles (paperback), and the cookbook The Wahls Protocol Cooking for Life: The Revolutionary Modern Paleo Plan to Treat All Chronic Autoimmune Conditions.
She conducts clinical trials that test the effect of nutrition and lifestyle interventions to treat MS and other progressive health problems. Learn more about Dr. Wahls' clinical trials here. She also teaches the public and medical community about the healing power of the Paleo diet and therapeutic lifestyle changes that restore health and vitality to our citizens.

She hosts a Wahls Protocol Seminar every August where anyone can learn how to implement the Protocol with ease and success. Follow her on Facebook (Terry Wahls MD) and on Twitter at @TerryWahls.

Books:	The Wahls Protocol: A Radical New Way to Treat All Chronic Autoimmune Conditions Using Paleo Principles
	Minding My Mitochondria 2nd Edition: How I overcame
	secondary progressive multiple sclerosis (MS) and
got out of	my wheelchair.
Website:	https://terrywahls.com/

Dr. Tommy Wood

Dr. Tommy Wood studied biochemistry at Cambridge University before earning a medical degree from Oxford University. He completed his foundation doctor training at St. Thomas' in London, and is now a PhD Fellow at the University of Oslo. The focus of his research is neonatal brain metabolism and developmental brain injury. Dr. Wood is the Chief Scientific Officer of the Physicians and Ancestral Health Society. He has researched and published on a broad range of topics, from biomarkers of sugar intake in obesity to the use of systems analysis to elucidate the multiple factors associated with chronic disease progression, with a special interest in Multiple Sclerosis. Dr. Wood is a health and performance coach with experience training athletes in a number of sports as well as helping patients manage disease symptoms through the use of both lifestyle modification and modern biochemical testing. He has a special interest in the multiple interacting genetic, psychosocial, environmental, and lifestyle factors that induce and exacerbate chronic disease. (description from Icelandic Health Symposium).

Dr. Jay Wortman, M.D.
(text from https://lowcarbconferences.com/jay-wortman-md/)

Dr. Jay Wortman has worked in family medicine, public health, medical administration and research. He has held senior management positions in

Health Canada in Ottawa and Vancouver.

For the past 15 years Dr. Wortman has worked with low-carbohydrate ketogentic diet in both the research and practice settings. One of his studies was the subject of the Canadian Broadcasting Corporation documentary film, "My Big Fat Diet". Dr. Wortman is a frequent presenter on the benefits of a low carbohydrate high fat diet at scientific meetings and continuing medical education events.

Dr. Wortman is a Clinical Assistant Professor in the Faculty of Medicine at the University of British Columbia and has been a member of the Scientific Advisory Board of Atkins Nutritionals Inc. Dr. Wortman currently practices in West Vancouver where he uses a low carb high fat diet for the treatment of metabolic and inflammatory conditions.

Website: http://www.drjaywortman.com/

___

William Yancy MD, MHS
Internal medicine doctor, obesity medicine specialist, researcher and Fellow of The Obesity Society and a diplomat of the American Board of Obesity Medicine

Dr. William Yancy has spent most of his career researching obesity and treatments for obesity. He is an associate professor of medicine at Duke University and a staff physician and a researcher at the Durham VA Medical Center.

He is also the director at Duke Diet and Fitness Center, an immersive, residential-style, comprehensive weight management program that serves patients from around the world who come to Duke for a week or longer to change their eating and activity lifestyles, lose weight, improve their health and learn strategies for long-term success.

Dr. Yancy has conducted multiple clinical trials investigating how different dietary and medicinal approaches affect body weight, cardiovascular risk and diabetes, with particular expertise regarding low-carbohydrate eating. He has also performed a number of studies examining innovative approaches toward improving adherence to lifestyle recommendations and other treatments. He has received several awards for his research and published over 100 peer-reviewed scientific articles.

He received his medical degree from East Carolina University and completed his residency at the University of Pittsburgh. He also has Masters in Health Sciences from Duke University.

Website: https://medicine.duke.edu/faculty/william-samuel-yancy-md

Chiropractic Doctors

Dr. Eric Berg D.C.

Eric Berg is a chiropractor who specializes in Health Ketosis™ and Intermittent Fasting. His clients have included senior officials in the U.S. government and the Justice Department, ambassadors, medical doctors, high-level executives of prominent corporations, scientists, engineers, professors, and other clients from all walks of life. Currently Dr. Berg no longer practices, but does full time education through social media, videos and conventions.

Books: The Healthy Keto Plan: Get Healthy, Lose Weight &
Feel Great

Website: www.drberg.com

Dr. Sten Ekberg D.C. -

Sten Anders Ekberg is a former decathlon athlete who competed in the 1992 Summer Olympics for Sweden and a Swedish decathlete National Record holder. Sten Ekberg won the Swedish Championship in both decathlon and heptathlon. Ekberg currently resides in the United States where he works as a chiropractor and nutritionist at his office Wellness For Life in Cumming, Georgia. — Wikipedia

Website: https://www.drekberg.com

Dr. Daniel Pompa D.C.

Dr. Pompa has established his coaching and teaching on a firm and proven conviction that the crisis of modern-day allopathic medicine is the sad result of physicians chasing symptoms with medication rather than addressing the root cause of disease. This even occurs within functional medicine. His approach to getting to the "upstream cause" is what separates him from others in allopathic as well as functional medicine. His clients receive coaching based on the fact that God created the human body with the ability to heal itself when interferences such as heavy metal toxicity, poor nutrition, and subluxations (whether physical, emotional or chemical) are removed. [description from his website]

Books: The Cellular Healing Diet

Website: http://www.drpompa.com

Dietitians and RNs

Amy Berger (description from her website)

Lives in the Durham, NC area, but works with clients all over the US and even internationally, via phone and Skype. She has a master's degree in human nutrition from the University of Bridgeport. She is also a Certified Nutrition Specialist (CNS). This designation requires a master's degree, passing a board exam, and accumulating 1000 hours of supervised clinical practice and other professional nutrition work. In this way, the requirements are similar to those for being a registered dietitian (RD), but the education programs are very different. She happen to also be a U.S. Air Force veteran, but that doesn't have much bearing on my nutrition career, except that I used my GI Bill to get the master's degree, so that was pretty nice.

She has been eating a low carbohydrate diet and learning about this way of eating for over 15 years. Her specific areas of interest include using low carb and ketogentic diets as nutritional therapies for diabetes (both type 2 and type 1), obesity, PCOS, migraines, acid reflux/GERD, cardiovascular disease, and neurological & neurodegenerative disorders (such as Alzheimer's, Parkinson's, multiple sclerosis, and epilepsy).

Books: The Alzheimer's Antidote: Using a Low-Carb, High-Fat Diet to Fight Alzheimer's Disease, Memory Loss, and Cognitive Decline.

Website: http://www.tuitnutrition.com/

Adele Hite

I came to rhetoric and communication from a Ph.D. program in nutritional epidemiology and a background in nutrition, dietetics, and public health. I was driven largely by frustration and questions I couldn't answer (or even figure out how to ask). I've been inspired and challenged by the theoretical frameworks offered by rhetoric and communication, and I have found my work going in directions I could not have envisioned previously. (description from her website)

Website: Adelehite.com

Resources
Vicky Kuriel - LCHF Dietician

Vicky Kuriel is a registered Australian Dietician and the co-founder of Acacia Health (http://acaciahealth.com.au). Her qualifications and experience cross the spectrum in the health, nutrition and fitness industries. She has 16 years experience in consulting, presenting, lecturing, training, instructing and writing and is recognised as a pioneer of Pilates in Australia.

Vicky is a proud proponent of a Low Carb, High fat lifestyle. Her beliefs, recommendations and dietary protocols may be contrary to the Australian Dietary guidelines however she has spent years engrossed in the health, fitness and nutrition industry researching, experimenting and fine-tuning. This research is on-going and an integral part of her practice today. She therefore stands strong on the LCHF, whole food, unprocessed, clean lifestyle recommendations… and loves sharing her passion for this way of living.

Feng-Yuan Liu - dietitian

Melbourne dietitian Feng-Yuan Liu has a Bachelor degree in Nutrition and Dietetics from Monash University as well as Post Graduate qualifications in Sports Nutrition through Sports Dietitians Australia, completed at the Australian Institute of Sport (AIS). She is also clinical dietitian founder and co-director of Metro Dietetics.

Feng-Yuan Liu is an Accredited Practicing Dietitian and one of a relatively rare but growing species: a dietitian who is a member of Dietitians Association of Australia (DAA) and brave enough to speak up publicly for LCHF (low-carbohydrate, high-fat) diets to treat obesity and diabetes.

She and her team at Metro Dietetics utilize up-to-date research to assist clients achieve results, as opposed to following Guidelines and dogma. She believes that nutritional science is a rapidly progressive science, and just following guidelines will not allow her clients to receive the best quality care that is available.

Feng-Yuan has now stepped into the role of creating and facilitating innovative programs for Metro Dietetics and The Keto Clinic, and

partnerships with other leaders in their field, to bring about a revolutionary change in the space of health and nutrition.
(description from Low carb down under)

Ali Miller, RD, LD, CDE

Description from:
ADAPT SAN ANTONIO TX - Low Carb Keto Living in the 21st Century

An integrative functional medicine practitioner with a background in naturopathic medicine. She is a Registered and Licensed Dietitian, Certified Diabetes Educator.

Ali has a contagious passion for food-as-medicine developing clinical protocols and virtual programs using nutrients and food as the foundation of treatment. Her approach is supported by up-to-date scientific research for a functional way to heal the body by addressing the root cause. Ali is a renowned expert in the ketogentic diet with over a decade of clinical results using a unique whole foods approach to a high fat low carb protocol. Ali's message has influenced the medical community with contributions to research studies and lectures to medical organizations and has impacted millions through media with television segments, print features, and her award winning podcast, Naturally Nourished. Ali's expertise can be accessed through her website: www.alimillerRD.com offering her blog, podcast, virtual learning, and access to her practice. Stay connected on instagram or facebook @alimillerRD

Website: www.alimillerRD.com

Books: Naturally Nourished: Food-as-Medicine for Optimal
         Health cookbook (2016),
                  The Anti-Anxiety Diet (2018),
                  The Anti-Anxiety Diet Cookbook (2019)

Lily Nichols - Registered Dietitian/Nutritionist, Certified Diabetes Educator

Lily's bestselling book, '*Real Food for Gestational Diabetes*' (and on-line course of the same name), presents a revolutionary nutrient-dense, lower carb diet for managing gestational diabetes. Her unique approach has not only helped tens of thousands of women manage their gestational diabetes (most without the need for blood sugar-lowering medication), but has also influenced nutrition policies internationally.

Lily's second book, *'Real Food for Pregnancy'*, is an evidence-based look at the gap between conventional prenatal nutrition guidelines and what's optimal for mother and baby. With over 930 citations, this is the most comprehensive text on prenatal nutrition to date.
(from lowcarbdownunder.com.au)

Books: Real Food for Gestational Diabetes
Real Food for Pregnancy

Website: www.LilyNicholsRDN.com

━━

Kelley Pound RN, CDE (description from her website)

I'm going to take a moment to introduce myself. My name is Kelley Pounds. I am a wife, mother, Registered Nurse and Certified Diabetes Educator by trade. I have battled my weight from childhood…attending Weight Watchers as early as age 10 (I've done Weight Watchers 4 times in my life). I've also tried other diets, like low fat, per-packaged food diets and calorie restricted diets, sometimes consuming as little as 500 calories a day in an effort to lose weight. They were all miserable failures and none contributed to good health.

Now in my early 40's, I was tired and fed up. My health was declining. I was pre-diabetic with elevated cholesterol and triglycerides, high blood pressure, acid reflux, poor mood and extreme low self esteem! My lack of energy was profound.

At the suggestion of my dad, himself a Type 2 diabetic who had lost 80 lbs and was managing his diabetes with a low carb lifestyle, I started to read, and thoroughly research this way of eating. As a nurse, it all made so much sense to me. I started to eliminate sugar and processed grains and starches, and started to replace them with real, whole foods and healthy sources of carbohydrates with increased emphasis on healthy fats. For the first time in years, I felt energetic, and the weight started melting off.

Website: https://lowcarbrn.wordpress.com

Franziska Spritzler

Franziska Spritzler is a registered dietitian, author and certified diabetes educator who takes a low-carb, real-food approach to diabetes, weight management and overall health. She lives in south Florida and has been following a low-carb lifestyle since early 2011. Franziska is also a freelance writer whose articles have been published on-line and in diabetes journals and magazines.

Books: The Low Carb Dietitian's Guide to Health and Beauty: How a Whole-Foods, Low-Carbohydrate Lifestyle Can Help You Look and Feel Better Than Ever

Autophagy: Body's Natural Intelligence for Anti-Aging and Healing - Intermittent Fasting for Weight Loss & Self-Cleansing: Healthy Eating

Website: http://www.lowcarbdietitian.com/

Caryn Zinn, PhD.

Caryn is an internationally-recognized leader and advocate of the whole food, low carbohydrate, healthy fat (LCHF) nutrition and lifestyle approach and its application to metabolic health and sports performance.

Caryn is an academic, an author and a registered dietitian, with over 20 years of consulting experience.

Website: https://www.carynzinn.co.nz/

Books: What The Fat? Fat's IN, Sugar's OUT
What The Fat? Sports Performance

Researchers and PhDs

Dr. Peter Ballerstedt - Agronomist

Peter Ballerstedt has the background and personality to help us bridge the knowledge gap between how we feed and raise our animals, and how we feed and raise ourselves! His fascinating story begins with understanding animal nutrition and food systems, but quickly transitioned to human nutrition as well after a personal health discovery. Since then, he has become a leading voice to promote a rational and science... (from Dietdoctor.com)

"Perhaps it is not the grain fed cattle but the grain fed people"

Dr. Jonny Bowden -

PhD in holistic nutrition and the board exams in nutrition for the American College of Nutrition, earning board certification and the CNS (Certified Nutrition Specialist) designation from the College's Certifying Board of Nutrition Specialists

Website: https://jonnybowden.com

Dr. Maryanne Demasi

Dr. Maryanne Demasi is a former medical scientist who completed her PhD in Medicine at the University of Adelaide. Her research focused on the pathology of Rheumatoid arthritis and potential therapies. Her innovative research has appeared in several internationally published medical journals.

Leaving her lab coat behind, Maryanne accepted a position as a political advisor and speech-writer for the South Australian Minister for Science and Information technology portfolios. She advised on issues concerning Intellectual Property and commercialization of research.

David Diamond PhD.

David M. Diamond is a professor in the Departments of Psychology and Molecular Pharmacology and Physiology at the University of South Florida and is a Research Career Scientist at the Tampa Veterans Hospital, where he has directed his research program on post-traumatic stress disorder (PTSD) and traumatic brain injury (TBI). He has also served as the Director of the USF Neuroscientist Collaborative program and is a Fellow at the American Institute of Stress and the International Stress and Behavior Society.

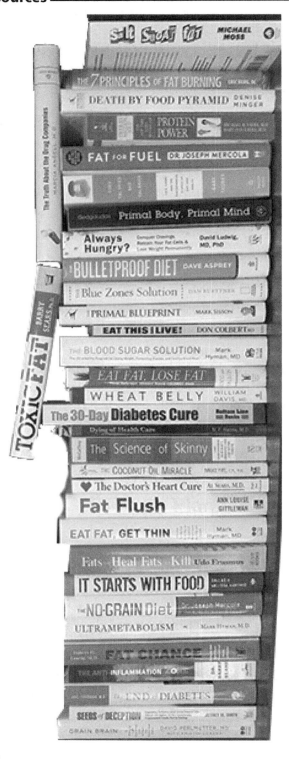

Some of the books I purchased for research while writing this book.

Books: Fat and Cholesterol Don't Cause Heart Attacks and Statins are Not The Solution

Mary G. Enig

Mary Gertrude Enig was a nutritionist and researcher known for her unconventional positions on the role saturated fats play in diet and health.
- Wikipedia

Books: Know Your Fats : The Complete Primer for Understanding the Nutrition of Fats, Oils and Cholesterol
Eat Fat, Lose Fat

Website: https://www.westonaprice.org

Dr. Zoe Harcome
A researcher, author, blogger and public speaker in the field of diet and health.

Books: The Diet Fix

Website: http://www.zoeharcombe.com

P.D. Mangan
P. D. (Dennis) Mangan has a background in microbiology and pharmacology. He lives in California, where he lifts weights in a run-down gym.

Books: Dumping Iron: How to Ditch This Secret Killer and Re claim Your Health

Stop the Clock: The Optimal Anti-Aging Strategy

Muscle Up: How Strength Training Beats Obesity, Cancer, and Heart Disease, and Why Everyone Should Do It

Smash Chronic Fatigue: A Concise, Science-Based Guide to

Sally Fallon Morell

The President of the Weston Price foundation. According to the WAPF, she received a B.A. in English from Stanford University and an M.A. in English from UCLA.

The foundation has seven board members and numerous honorary board members, most of whom have medical or nutritional qualifications

Books: Nourishing Fats: Why We Need Animal Fats for Health and Happiness
Nourishing Diets: How Paleo, Ancestral and Traditional Peoples Really Ate

Ivor Cummins

From Low Carb Breckenridge 2018 Conference:
Ivor originally completed a Chemical Engineering degree in 1990 (Biochemical Stream, BE(Chem) CEng MIEI, followed by over 25 years in corporate technical leadership and management positions. Ivor's particular specialty was leading teams in complex problem-solving scenarios. Following less-than-ideal blood test results, he was unable to get solutions

from the doctors he consulted. He thus embarked on an intense period of biochemical research into the science of human metabolism. Ivor intensively studied the mechanisms and primary drivers of elevated GGT and Serum Ferritin. This quickly led to an investigation of general causes of inflammation and dyslipidemia. Within eight weeks Ivor had resolved and optimized all of his blood test metrics. Also, he had shed nearly 15kg of body fat with relative ease. As the journey became a fixation he went on to analyze over 200 related papers and studies carried out over the past 5 decades and before.

Book: Eat Rich, Live Long: Mastering the Low-Carb & Keto Spectrum for Weight Loss and Longevity

Website: https://thefatemperor.com

Gary Taubes

Gary Taubes is an investigative science and health journalist and co-founder of the non-profit Nutrition Science Initiative (NuSI.org). He is the author of *Why We Get Fat and What to Do About It* and *Good Calories, Bad Calories (The Diet Delusion in the UK)*. Taubes is the recipient of a Robert Wood Johnson Foundation Investigator Award in Health Policy Research, and has won numerous other awards for his journalism. These include the International Health Reporting Award from the Pan American Health Organization and the National Association of Science Writers Science in Society Journalism Award, which he won in 1996, 1999 and 2001. (He is the first print journalist to win this award three times.) Taubes graduated from Harvard College in 1977 with an S.B. degree in applied physics, and received an M.S. degree in engineering from Stanford University (1978) and in journalism from Columbia University (1981).

Books: Why We Get Fat: And What to Do About It
                The Case Against Sugar
                Good Calories, Bad Calories

Website: https://garytaubes.com

Nina Teicholz

Nina Teicholz is an investigative science journalist and leader in nutrition reporting who is challenging the conventional wisdom on dietary fat–particularly, whether saturated fat causes heart disease and whether fat really makes you fat. The New York Times bestselling author of *The Big Fat Surprise*. Teicholz also serves as Executive Director of The Nutrition Coalition, an independent non-profit group that promotes evidence-based nutrition policy. She is one of a new generation of researchers arguing that diets lower in carbohydrates are a scientifically sound approach for reversing nutrition-related diseases. (description from her website)

Books: The Big Fat Surprise: Why Butter, Meat and Cheese Belong in a Healthy Diet
Website: https://ninateicholz.com/

Dave Feldman

Software engineer and entrepreneur. He began a Low Carb, High Fat diet in April 2015 and has since learned everything he could about it with special emphasis on cholesterol given his lipid numbers spiked substantially after going on the diet. As an engineer, he spotted a pattern in the lipid system that's very similar to distributed objects in networks.

He has since learned quite a bit on the subject both through research and experimentation which has revealed some very powerful data. With this new general theory, He shifted around his cholesterol more than anyone else in the world without any drugs or special supplements of any kind.

Website: https://cholesterolcode.com/

Mikhaila Peterson - Blogger and founder of the Lion Diet

I promote an unusual diet that has allowed me to get off of over 10 medications and put my several, seemingly incurable, life-long diseases into complete remission. By the age of 22 I was diagnosed with juvenile rheumatoid arthritis (age 7), depression (age 12), bipolar type II, idiopathic hypersomnia, lyme disease, psoriasis, and dyshidrotic eczema. They're all in remission with strict dietary adherence. I have a healthy daughter, I have my life back and I've seen hundreds of others have similar remissions. This lifestyle is centered around a diet consisting solely of beef, salt, and water supported with numerous health and wellness practices (some rather unorthodox). I tell my story to help people realize that they shouldn't give up on their health, no matter how hopeless it may seem, and that it is their responsibility to fix themselves. Bodies have an amazing capacity to heal, if we just let them, but figuring out how to do that and pursuing it is up to you.

Website: https://mikhailapeterson.com

Mark Sisson

Health and fitness expert Mark Sisson is the bestselling author of The Primal Blueprint and several other Primal Blueprint-branded books, and one of the leading voices of the burgeoning Evolutionary Health Movement. His blog, MarksDailyApple.com, has paved the way for Primal enthusiasts to challenge conventional wisdom's diet and exercise principles and take personal responsibility for their health and well-being.

Book: The Primal Blueprint

Website: https://www.marksdailyapple.com/

Websites:
(Only a few of the many great sites)

Dietdoctor.com

Our trusted guides are written or reviewed by medical doctors, and based on science. To stay unbiased we show no ads, take no industry money and sell no products. Instead we're funded by the people, via an optional membership.

JumpstartMD.com

Our personalized science-based program is medically designed by Stanford-trained physicians and based on proven nutritional science. We combine leading-edge research, quantified biometrics, and physician supervision to create safe and effective weight loss programs.

https://www.lowcarbusa.org

https://www.virtahealth.com/

Weight loss without low-calorie diets or surgery Our patients quickly lose clinically significant amounts of weight, and are able to sustain or improve upon their initial losses. After 1 year, patients achieved an average weight loss of 30lbs.

https://healclinics.com/

A personalized, guided, uncomplicated ketogentic path to putting obesity, pre-diabetes and type 2 diabetes in remission

https://peterattiamd.com/

Peter Attia explores strategies and tactics to increase lifespan, health span, and well-being, and optimize cognitive, physical, and emotional health.

https://www.ketogenicdocs.com

Connecting you with Health practitioners that support a ketogentic lifestyle.

https://www.nutritioncoalition.us/

The Nutrition Coalition (TNC) is a 501(c)(3) non-profit, non-partisan educational organization, founded in 2015, with the primary goal of ensuring that U.S. nutrition policy is based on rigorous scientific evidence. We promote the importance of adopting a state-of-the-art scientific process for ensuring evidence-based nutrition policy.

TNC is actively building a broad and diverse coalition of scientists, health-care practitioners, researchers, policy makers, and concerned citizens to fight nutrition-related chronic diseases in America through rigorous science, education, and effective communication. We invite you to join us. Together, we can change the Dietary Guidelines for Americans, improve public health, and reduce related medical costs for generations to come.

Https://thincs.org/

International Network of Cholestrol skeptics

smashthefat.com

https://price-pottenger.org

The Price-Pottenger Nutrition Foundation is a U.S. 501 non-profit organization established "to teach the public and professionals about foods, lifestyle habits, healing modalities, and environmental practices that can help people attain vibrant health." Founded in 1952, it was first known as the Santa Barbara Medical Research Foundation and later renamed the Weston A. - Wikipedia

Books (just a few)

(Descriptions of the books are from the Amazon Website)

The Fat Revolution - Christine Cronau

Discover the story behind the biggest scam of the 21st century. The Fat Revolution is a fascinating and controversial disclosure, debunking 'conventional wisdom' about what constitutes a healthy lifestyle and diet. This book is an invaluable look into what makes us fat and the real cause of heart disease.

Learn why fat can't make you fat, exercise is unnecessary for weight-loss, saturated fat is NOT the demon it has been portrayed to be, and why, in fact, low-fat diets are fattening.

Nutrition and Physical Degeneration. - Dr. Weston A. Price DDS

An epic study demonstrating the importance of whole food nutrition, and the degeneration and destruction that comes from a diet of processed foods.

Pure, White and Deadly - John Yudkin - Penguin Books

Pure, White, and Deadly, first published in 1972, and was one of the first scientists to claim that sugar was a major cause of obesity and heart disease.

The Big Fat Surprise: Why Butter, Meat and Cheese Belong in a Healthy Diet - Nina Teicholz - Simon & Schuster

Nina Teicholz is an investigative science journalist and author as well as an advocate for evidence-based nutrition policy. Her work has appeared in The New York Times, The Wall Street Journal, The Independent, The Atlantic, and The New Yorker, among other places. She grew up in Berkeley, California, and now lives in New York.

The Sugar Fix: The High-Fructose Fallout That Is Making You Fat and Sick - Richard Johnson and Tim Gowe - Rodale Books

In The Sugar Fix, Dr. Richard Johnson, who oversees a pioneering research program, reports on discoveries about how fructose impacts the body—and directly connects the American obesity epidemic to a frightening escalation in our fructose consumption.

It comes as no surprise that the sugar is found in processed foods like candy, baked goods, canned foods, and frozen meals in the form of high-fructose corn syrup, but it is also hidden in less obvious foods like peanut butter, egg products, and soups. Many fruits and vegetables contain high levels of it naturally. Dr. Johnson shows how to cut way back on the sweetener by making effective substitutions. The daily meal plans included here contain no more than 25 grams of fructose, one-quarter of the amount the average American now ingests.

Big Fat Lies: How The Diet Industry Is Making You Sick, Fat & Poor
- David Gillespie - Penguin

'Diets and exercise won't help us lose weight. Vitamins and minerals are a waste of money and sometimes downright dangerous. Sugar makes us fat and sick. And polyunsaturated fat gives us cancer and works with sugar to give us heart disease. This book exists because I desperately hope that with a little knowledge we can all vote with out feet and change the rules of the game before the game kills us.' For decades we've been told to eat less, exercise more, eat less saturated fat, eat more polyunsaturated oils, and take vitamin and omega-3 fatty acid supplements. For decades this is what we've done, but the rates of obesity, heart disease, type 2 diabetes, dementia and cancer have never been higher. The real culprits, David Gillespie tells us, are sugar and polyunsaturated oils. Analyzing the latest scientific evidence, he shows us why the outlines a plan to avoid them both without missing out or 'dieting'. Gillespie exposes the powerful role the multi billion-dollar food, health and diet industries have played in promoting the health messages we follow or feel guilty about not following. Discovering the truth about diets, exercise, supplements and processed food is your first step towards improved health, greater happiness and a longer life for you and your family. 'Gillespie is an informed and entertaining writer who makes his subject fascinating, and inspires with his passion and logic.' G MAGAZINE

Eat Fat, Lose Fat: The Healthy Alternative to Trans Fats
- Sally Fallon & Mary G. Enig

A diet and nutrition book from a new perspective, dispelling the myth that dietary fat is bad and shows that these saturated fats like coconut oil, red meat, and butter are actually essential to weight loss and health.

Based on over two decades of research, Eat Fat, Lose Fat flouts conventional wisdom by revealing that vegetable oils (such as corn and soybean) are in large part responsible for our national obesity and health crisis, while healthy fats such as those found in coconut oil may actually be the secret to long-term wellness.

Filled with delicious coconut oil-based recipes, this book features three programs that help you get started eating healthy fats to lose weight and achieve good health for a lifetime

---

Fat and Cholesterol Don't Cause Heart Attacks and Statins are Not The Solution - by Paul J. Rosch MD (Author), Zoë Harcombe PhD (Author), Malcolm Kendrick MD (Author), Uffe Ravnskov MD PhD (Author), Fred A. Kummerow PhD (Author), Harumi Okuyama PhD (Author), & 15 more

As will be seen, no studies support the notion that restricting fat reduces coronary morbidity or mortality. More importantly, government recommendations mandating low fat diets are likely the cause of the escalating epidemic of obesity and type 2 diabetes. Several chapters detail the panoply of significant adverse health effects of statins that have been ignored or suppressed in reports of drug company sponsored trials. These include promoting the development of coronary atherosclerosis and congestive failure. In addition, the putative benefits of statins are clearly unrelated to lowering LDL or cholesterol, but rather anti-inflammatory and especially anticoagulant activities. This clotting or "atherothrombotic" hypothesis appears to explain all of the factors known to cause or protect against coronary heart disease. Other chapters by THINCS members discuss the role of infections and sulfur deficiency, and the numerous ways data are doctored to hype the benefits and minimize the dangers of statins. All of these contributions expose the fallacies of the lipid hypothesis, which was called "the greatest scientific deception of this century, perhaps of any century" by the distinguished nutritionist George Mann, former Co-Director of the Framingham Study.

The Dark Side of Statins - The Wonder of Cholestrol
- Dr. Duane Graveline

This is Dr. Duane Graveline's fourth and final book on statin drugs. This new (August 2017) and expanded edition of The Dark Side of Statins completes the series. All four of his statin books are equally informative, but he considered this to be both the best and the most important of his works. The final chapter is a first-hand account of Dr Graveline's last weeks and days and the official causes of his death. The full range of statin side effects includes cognitive dysfunction, behavioral and emotional disorders, chronic nerve and muscle damage and an ALS-like neuromuscular degenerative process, as major categories of damage. Thousands of statin users, like myself, have been afflicted with peripheral neuropathies with a tendency to be resistant to all traditional medical treatment. Statins inhibit not only dolichols, corrupting our DNA damage correction, but CoQ10 as well, increasing our damage load. Predictably the inevitable effect is increased mitochondrial DNA damage — considered by many authorities to be the mechanism of our aging process as well as that of many chronic diseases. Many of the statin side effects are permanent and weakness and fatigue are common complaints. Many statin victims say that abruptly, almost in the blink of an eye, they have become old people. Statins block the synthesis of CoQ10 and dolichols, thereby contributing directly to the premature common chronic ills of aging. Since this involves normal physiologic processes, it is silent. By the time we become aware of it, it is already far too late and the damage has been done to those susceptible. This, in my judgment, is the truly Dark Side of Statins.

This is Dr Duane Graveline's fourth and final book on statins

---

Lies My Doctor Told Me Second Edition: Medical Myths That Can Harm Your Health - Dr. Ken Berry M.D.

This book will teach you:
- Facts doctors are taught to think about nutrition and other preventative health measures and how they should be thinking
- Story of how the food pyramid and MyPlate came into existence and why they should change
- Facts about fat intake and heart health
- Truth about the effects of whole wheat on the human body
- Role of dairy in your diet
- Truth about salt - friend or foe?
- Dangers and benefits of hormone therapy
- New information about inflammation and how it should be viewed by doctors
- Come out of the darkness and let Ken Berry be your guide to optimal health and harmony

The Statin Damage Crisis - Dr. Duane Graveline M.D.

Tens of thousands of people have been victims of a huge array of statin drugs side effects, ranging from permanent cognitive dysfunction and severe personality change to disabilities from permanent peripheral neuropathy, permanent myopathy and chronic muscular degeneration. It has been reported that muscle pain cases frequently become permanent and many neurologists now regard statin neuropathy as predictably resistant to traditional treatment.

In addition to the crisis of thousands of people disabled by statin associated neuro-muscular problems is the fact that many physicians still remain unaware that statins can even do this. Then there is the crisis of patients being forced into taking a statin because not to do so would result in having to find a new doctor.

The Statin Damage Crisis looks at how statins work, the importance of cholesterol in the body, inflammation and atherosclerosis, anti-inflammatory alternatives to statins, serious side effects of statins, plus dietary supplements of possible benefit to those taking statins or that were forced to stop taking a statin due to unpleasant and even disabling side effects.

The Complete Guide to Fasting: Heal Your Body Through Intermittent, Alternate-Day, and Extended Fasting by Jimmy Moore, Dr. Jason Fung, et al.

The Complete Guide to Fasting explains:

- Why fasting is actually good for health
- Who can benefit from fasting (and who won't)
- The history of fasting
- The various ways to fast: intermittent, alternate-day, and extended fasting
- What to expect when starting to fast
- How to track progress while fasting
- The weight loss effects of fasting
- How to ward off potential negative effects from fasting

Not by bread alone - Eating meat and fat for stay Lean and Healthy by Vilhjalmur Stefansson

The author details his experiment in extreme nutrition. This famous book extols the virtues of meat in the human diet.

There are many more excellent resources for your own research.

The Vegetarian Myth: Food, Justice, and Sustainability by Lierre Keith

Part memoir, nutritional primer, and political manifesto, this controversial examination exposes the destructive history of agriculture—causing the devastation of prairies and forests, driving countless species extinct, altering the climate, and destroying the topsoil—and asserts that, in order to save the planet, food must come from within living communities. In order for this to happen, the argument champions eating locally and sustainably and encourages those with the resources to grow their own food. Further examining the question of what to eat from the perspective of both human and environmental health, the account goes beyond health choices and discusses potential moral issues from eating—or not eating—animals. Through the deeply personal narrative of someone who practiced veganism for 20 years, this unique exploration also discusses alternatives to industrial farming, reveals the risks of a vegan diet, and explains why animals belong on ecologically sound farms.
(description from Amazon.com)

How Nature Cures: Comprising a New System of Hygiene; Also the Natural Food of Man; a Statement of the Principal Arguments Against the Use of Bread, ... Pulses, Potatoes, and All Other Starch Foods - Emmet Densmore published 1892

(Description from Amazon)
This work has been selected by scholars as being culturally important, and is part of the knowledge base of civilization as we know it. This work was reproduced from the original artifact, and remains as true to the original work as possible. Therefore, you will see the original copyright references, library stamps (as most of these works have been housed in our most important libraries around the world), and other notations in the work.

This work is in the public domain in the United States of America, and possibly other nations. Within the United States, you may freely copy and distribute this work, as no entity (individual or corporate) has a copyright on the body of the work.

You can read the book on-line for free:
https://archive.org/details/ hownaturecuresc01densgoog/page/n6/mode/2up

A few Movies

These movies are great documentaries of the LCHF lifestyle and the dangers of certain drugs and toxic sugar

Carb-Loaded: A Culture Dying to Eat
(description from amazon.com)

Carb-Loaded: A Culture Dying to Eat is a chronicle of the things its writer and director, Lathe Poland, learned after he was diagnosed with Type 2 diabetes. He sought to find out why he got sick because he didn't fit the classic picture of an adult-onset diabetes sufferer. In the film, he searches out why America's modern food culture is killing us. There is an upside, and a lot that can be done!

Cereal Killers - Don't fear the fat
http://www.cerealkillersmovie.com/
(description from DietDoctor.com)

What if everything you knew about sports nutrition was wrong? What if there was no need for carbs or sports drinks when you exercise? What if you could – in fact – break records rowing across the Pacific Ocean without it? The documentary Cereal Killers follows Donal O'Neill, who tries to avoid walking in his father's footsteps (with heart disease) by eating a high-fat diet.

The hour-long movie follows his experiences during four weeks of high-fat dieting, including careful medical examinations. Don't miss the surprised lab technician 48 minutes into the movie. Donal's basic metabolic rate increased according to the examinations, which the technician says he's never seen before and can't figure out why it happened. Perhaps he needs to read up a little.

In the movie we can also see Professor Tim Noakes from South Africa, Dr. Briffa from England and an Australian cricket team.

Fat Fiction
Forget Everything You've Been Told About Fat.

What if everything we've been told about saturated fat is fiction? And what if the "low fat, heart healthy" diet represents one of the most damaging public health recommendations in the history of our country? FAT FICTION (formerly known as BIG FAT LIE) is a film that questions decades of diet advice insisting that saturated fats are bad for us. Along the way, we'll reveal the lies we've been told about fats, learn what fats are good, what fats are bad, and what we can do to reclaim our health.

Fat Head

Comedian and health writer Tom Naughton replies to the "Super Size Me" crowd by losing weight on a fat-laden fast-food diet while demonstrating that nearly everything we've been told about obesity and healthy eating is wrong.

Fat Chance - Is Butter The New Super food?
(description from DietDoctor.com)

Is it possible to ride a pushbike across the Australian continent (2,100 miles / 3,400 km) without eating carbohydrates?

The Perfect Human Diet
C.J. Hunt

The Perfect Human Diet is the unprecedented global exploration for a solution to our epidemic of overweight, obesity and diet-related diseases

- the #1 killer in America. This film, by broadcast journalist C.J. Hunt, bypasses current dietary group-think by exploring modern dietary science, previous historical findings, ancestral native diets and the emerging field of human dietary evolution - revealing for the first time, the authentic human diet. Film audiences finally can see what our species truly needs for optimal health and are given a practical template based on scientific facts. Written by C. J. Hunt

[I vehemently disagree with their evolutionary explanations]

Appendix D

Bibliography

Bibliography

Autophagy: How to Combine Intermittent Fasting and Nobel-Prize Winning Science for Rapid Weight Loss, Reducing Inflammation, and Promoting Long-Term Health - Thomas Hawthorn - Amazon

AUTOPHAGY: Body's Natural Intelligence for Anti-Aging and Healing – Intermittent Fasting for Weight Loss & Self-Cleansing (Healthy Eating Book 2) - Frances Spritzler - Amazon

The Blue Zones Solution - Eating and Living Like the World's Healthiest People - Dan Buettner - National Geographic

The Bulletproof Diet - Dave Asprey - Rodale Press

The Carnivore Diet With Intermittent Fasting by Michael D. Kaiser

Darwin's Black Box: The Biochemical Challenge to Evolution - Michael Behe - Simon and Schuster

Death by Food Pyramid: How Shoddy Science, Sketchy Politics and Shady Special Interests Ruined Your Health - Denise Minger - Primal Nutrition, Inc.

Deep Nutrition - Catherine Shanahan M.D. - Flatiron Books

Dying of Health Care - How the System Harms Americans Physcially and Financially, and How to Change It - N.F. Hanna, M.D. Copernicus Healthcare

Diabetes Epidemic and You - Dr. Joesph Kraft - Trafford Publishing

Diabetes Unpacked: Just Science and Sense, No Sugar Coating - by Prof Tim Noakes, Fung MD, Jason, Nina Teicholz , Kendrick MD, Malcolm, Harcombe PhD, Zoë, Cywes MD, Robert - Columbus Publishing Ltd

Eat Fat, Get Thin - Mark Hyman, M.D. - Little Brown

Eat Fat and Grow Slim Richard Mackarness, Zelma Mackenzie - Harper Collins Publishers

Eat Fat, Lose Fat - Dr. Mary Enig, Sally Fallon - Hudson Street Press

Eat Meat and Stop Jogging - Mike Sheredan - Lean Living Inc.

Eat to Beat Disease: The New Science of How Your Body Can Heal Itself - William Li - Grand Central Publishing;

Fat Chance - Robert H. Lustig, M.D. - Hudson Street Press

Fat and Cholesterol Don't Cause Heart Attacks and Statins are Not The Solution - Rosch MD, Paul J. (Author), Harcombe PhD, Zoë (Author), Kendrick MD, Malcolm (Author), Ravnskov MD PhD, Uffe & more - Columbus Publishing Ltd

Fat for Fuel - Dr. Joseph Mercola - Hay House Inc.

320

Fat Heals Sugar Kills - Dr. Bruce Fife - Piccadilly Books, Ltd.

The Fat Switch - Richard J. Johnson M.D. - Mercola.com

Food Rules - Catherine Shanahan M.D. - Big Box Books

Good Calories, Bad Calories - Gary Taubes - Anchor Books

Grain Brain - David Perlmutter, M.D. - Little Brown

Gut-Brain Secrets, Good Food, Bad Food - R.D. Lee - Amazon

Gut-Brain Secrets, R.D. Lee

Health and Vitality Truth - Dr. Luan Pho - Amazon

Ignore the Awkward - Uffe Ravinskov -

It Starts With Food - Dallas and Melissa Hartwig - Victory Belt Publishing

Just Tell Me What To Do - Kevin Davis PA-C - Amazon

Leptin Resistance - Dr. Nick Hibbert - Amazon

Know Your Fats - Dr. Mary Enig - Bethesda Press

Lies My Doctor Told Me Second Edition: Medical Myths That Can Harm Your Health - Ken Berry M.D. - Victory Belt Publishing

Live it Not Diet - Mike Sheridan - Living Lean Inc.

Mighty Mito - Dr. Susanne Bennett - Wellness For Life Press

My Life With The Eskimo - Vilhjalmur Stefansson - Macmillan Company

The Modern Nutritional Diseases: and How to Prevent Them - Alice Ottoboni, Ph.D., Fred Ottoboni, M.P.H., Ph.D.

The No-Grain Diet, Conquer Carbohydrate Addition and Stay Slim for Life - Dr. Joseph Mercola - Dutton

Nutrition and Physical Degeneration - W.A Price - Keats

Principia Ketogenica: Low Carbohydrate And Ketogenic Diets - Compendium Of Science Literature On The Benefits - Ash simmonds

Protein Power - Drs Michael and Mary Dan Eades - Bantam

The Primal Blueprint - Reprogram your genes for effortless weight loss, vibrant health, and boundless energy - Mark Sisson - Primal Nutrition

Primal Body Primal Mind - Beyond the Paleo Diet for Total Health and a Longer Life - Nora T. Gedgaudas, CNS,CNT - Healing Arts Press

Pure White and Deadly - John Yudkin - Penguin Books

Bibliography

https://archive.org/details/PureWhiteAndDeadly/page/n1

Salt Sugar Fat: How the Food Giants Hooked Us - Michael Moss - Random House

Seeds of Deception - Jeffery M. Smith - Yes Books

Signature in the Cell: DNA and the Evidence for Intelligent Design - Stephen C. Meyer - Harper Collins Publishers

Smart Fat: Eat More Fat. Lose More Weight. Get Healthy Now. - Masley M.D, Steven, Jonny Bowen - HarperOne

The Statin Damage Crisis - Duane Graveline MD - Spacedoc Media LLC

The Banting Pocket Guide - Tim Noakes - Penguin

The Calorie Myth: How to Eat More, Exercise Less, Lose Weight, and Live Better by Jonathan Bailor

The Case Against Sugar - Gary Taubes - Alfred Knopf

The Great Cholesterol Con: The Truth About What Really Causes Heart Disease and How to Avoid It - Malcolm Kendrick - John Blake Publishing

The Cholesterol Myths - Exposing the Fallacy that Saturated Fat and Cholesterol Cause Heart Disease - Uffe Ravnskov M.D. - Pragmatic Press

The Great Cholesterol Myth: Why Lowering Your Cholesterol Won't Prevent Heart Disease-and the Statin-Free Plan That Will - Jonny Bowden and Stephen Sinatra - Fair Winds Press

The Coconut Oil Miracle - Bruce Fife, C.N., N.D. - Avery (Penguin Group)

The Diabetes Code: Prevent and Reverse Type 2 Diabetes Naturally - Dr. Jason Fung and Nina Teicholz - Greystone Books

The Master Antioxidant Gluathione - Jeffrey Sutton - Amazon

The Mother of All Antioxidants: How Health Gurus are Misleading You and What You Should Know about Glutathione - Joey Lott - Amazon

Mysterious Epigenome - Woodward and Gills - Kregel Publications

The Seven Daughters of Eve - Bryan Sykes - W.W. Norton

The Truth About the Drug Companies: How They Deceive Us and What to Do About It - Dr. Marcia Angell - Random House Trade

Traditional Nutrition - Ben Hirshberg

Tripping over the Truth: How the Metabolic Theory of Cancer Is Overturning One of Medicine's Most Entrenched Paradigms - by Travis Christofferson

Trust Us We're Experts: How Industry Manipulates Science and Gambles with Your Future - Sheldon Rampton and John Stauber - TarcherPerigee

Ultra Metabolism - Mark Hyman, M.D. - Scribner

What The Fat - G. Schofield, Dr. C. Zinn, Craig Rodger - Real Food Pub

Why we get fat - Gary Taubes - Anchor Books

Wheat Belly - Dr. William Davis - Rodale Books

The Newer Knowledge Of Nutrition - The Use of Food For The Preservation Of Vitality and Health - 1918 - E.V. McCollum

Reference:

Netter's Internal Medicine - Runge and Greganti - Saunders

An Introduction to Chemistry for Biology Students - George Sackheim - Benjamin Cummins

Principles of Internal Medicine - McGraw Hill

The Human Body in Health and Disease - Wolters Kluwer - Health

Steadmans Medical Dictionary - Williams and Wilkins

The Merck Manual - MSD

Cellular and Molecular Immunology - Abbs and Lichtman - Saunders

Molecular Biology - Turner, Mclennan, Bates and White - Taylor & Francis

Structure & Function of the Body - Thirodbeau & Patton - Mosby

Genetics In Medicine - Nussbaum, McInnes, Willard - Saunders

Williams Textbook of Endocrinology - Wilson & Foster - Saunders

Cell Physiology Source Book - Sperelakis - Academic Press

Endocrine Physiology - Susan P. Porterfield - Mosby - Elsevier Science

Made in the USA
Middletown, DE
25 March 2023

27668019R00189